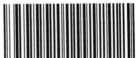

The Pharmacy Technician's Pocket Drug Reference

The Pharmacy Technician's Pocket Drug Reference

5th Edition

Joyce A. Generali, BPharm, MS, FASHP
Director, Drug Information Center
University of Kansas Medical Center
Kansas City, Kansas
Clinical Professor
University of Kansas School of Pharmacy
Lawrence, Kansas

American Pharmacists Association
Improving medication use. Advancing patient care.
APhA
Washington, D.C.

Editor: Nancy Tarleton Landis
Layout and Graphics: Michele Danoff
Cover Design: Scott Neitzke, APhA Creative Services

© 2009 by the American Pharmacists Association
Published by the American Pharmacists Association,
1100 15th Street, N.W., Suite 400, Washington, DC 20005-1707
www.pharmacist.com

APhA was founded in 1852 as the American Pharmaceutical Association.

To comment on this book via e-mail, send your message to the publisher at
aphabooks@aphanet.org.

Library of Congress Cataloging-in-Publication Data

Generali, Joyce A.
  The pharmacy technician's pocket drug reference / Joyce A. Generali.
— 5th ed.
    p. ; cm.
  Includes index.
  ISBN 978-1-58212-123-9
  1. Pharmacy technicians--Handbooks, manuals, etc. 2.
Drugs--Handbooks, manuals, etc. I. American Pharmacists Association.
II. Title.
  [DNLM: 1. Pharmaceutical Preparations—administration & dosage—
Handbooks. 2. Pharmacists' Aides—Handbooks. QV 735 G326p 2009]

  RS122.95.G464 2009
  615'.1--dc22

                        2008043654

How to Order This Book

Online: www.pharmacist.com
By phone: 800-878-0729 (770-280-0085 from outside the United States).
VISA®, MasterCard®, and American Express® cards accepted

GENERAL USES:
Hypertension, heart failure, left ventricular dysfunction, diabetic renal dysfunction

DOSAGE FORMS:
Tablets: 12.5 mg, 25 mg, 50 mg, 100 mg

CAPTOPRIL/HCTZ
KAP toe pril/hye droe klor oh THYE a zide

TRADE NAME(S):
Capozide

THERAPEUTIC CLASS:
Antihypertensive/diuretic

GENERAL USES:
Hypertension

DOSAGE FORMS:
Tablets: 25 mg/15 mg, 50 mg/15 mg, 25 mg/25 mg, 50 mg/25 mg

CARBAMAZEPINE
kar ba MAZ e peen

TRADE NAME(S):
Tegretol, Epitol, Equetro

THERAPEUTIC CLASS:
Anticonvulsant

GENERAL USES:
Seizures, trigeminal neuralgia

DOSAGE FORMS:
Chewable tablets: 100 mg; Tablets: 200 mg; Extended-release tablets: 100 mg, 200 mg, 400 mg; Extended-release capsules: 100 mg, 200 mg, 300 mg; Suspension: 100 mg/5 mL

CARBENICILLIN
kar ben i SIL in

TRADE NAME(S):
Geocillin

THERAPEUTIC CLASS:
Anti-infective

GENERAL USES:
Bacterial infections

DOSAGE FORMS:
Tablets: 382 mg

CARBIDOPA/LEVODOPA/ENTACAPONE
kar bi DOE pa/lee voe DOE pa/en TA ka pone

TRADE NAME(S):
Stalevo

THERAPEUTIC CLASS:
Antiparkinson agent

GENERAL USES:
Parkinson's disease

DOSAGE FORMS:
Tablets: 12.5 mg/50 mg/200 mg, 25 mg/100 mg/200 mg, 37.5 mg/150 mg/200 mg

CARISOPRODOL
kar i soe PROE dole

TRADE NAME(S):
Soma

THERAPEUTIC CLASS:
Skeletal muscle relaxant

GENERAL USES:
Musculoskeletal
conditions

DOSAGE FORMS:
Tablets: 250 mg, 350 mg

CARTEOLOL (OCULAR)
KAR tee oh lole

TRADE NAME(S):
Ocupress

THERAPEUTIC CLASS:
Ocular agent

GENERAL USES:
Glaucoma/ocular
hypertension

DOSAGE FORMS:
Ophthalmic solution: 1%

CARTEOLOL (ORAL)
KAR tee oh lole

TRADE NAME(S):
Cartrol

THERAPEUTIC CLASS:
Antihypertensive

GENERAL USES:
Hypertension

DOSAGE FORMS:
Tablets: 2.5 mg, 5 mg

CARVEDILOL
KAR ve dil ole

TRADE NAME(S):
Coreg, Coreg CR

THERAPEUTIC CLASS:
Antihypertensive,
cardiac agent

GENERAL USES:
Hypertension, CHF

DOSAGE FORMS:
Tablets: 3.125 mg,
6.25 mg, 12.5 mg, 25 mg;
Extended-release capsules:
10 mg, 20 mg, 40 mg,
80 mg

CASPOFUNGIN ACETATE
kas poe FUN jin

TRADE NAME(S):
Cancidas

THERAPEUTIC CLASS:
Antifungal

GENERAL USES:
Refractory aspergillosis
infection

DOSAGE FORMS:
Injection: 50 mg, 70 mg

CEFACLOR
SEF a klor

TRADE NAME(S):
Ceclor

THERAPEUTIC CLASS:
Anti-infective

GENERAL USES:
Bacterial infections

DOSAGE FORMS:
Capsules: 250 mg,
500 mg; Extended-release
tablets: 375 mg, 500 mg;
Suspension: 125 mg/

5 mL, 187 mg/5 mL,
250 mg/5 mL, 375 mg/
5 mL; Chewable tablets:
125 mg, 187 mg, 250 mg,
350 mg

CEFADROXIL
sef a DROKS il
TRADE NAME(S):
Duricef
THERAPEUTIC CLASS:
Anti-infective
GENERAL USES:
Bacterial infections
DOSAGE FORMS:
Capsules: 500 mg;
Tablets: 1 g; Suspension:
125 mg/5 mL,
250 mg/5 mL,
500 mg/5 mL

CEFAMANDOLE
sef a MAN dole
TRADE NAME(S):
Mandol
THERAPEUTIC CLASS:
Anti-infective
GENERAL USES:
Bacterial infections
DOSAGE FORMS:
Injection: 1 g, 2 g

CEFAZOLIN
sef A zoe lin
TRADE NAME(S):
Ancef, Kefzol
THERAPEUTIC CLASS:
Anti-infective

GENERAL USES:
Bacterial infections
DOSAGE FORMS:
Injection: 250 mg, 500 mg,
1 g, 5 g, 10 g, 20 g

CEFDINIR
SEF di ner
TRADE NAME(S):
Omnicef
THERAPEUTIC CLASS:
Anti-infective
GENERAL USES:
Bacterial infections
DOSAGE FORMS:
Capsules: 300 mg;
Suspension: 125 mg/
5 mL

CEFDITOREN PIVOXIL
sef di TOR en pye VOKS il
TRADE NAME(S):
Spectracef
THERAPEUTIC CLASS:
Anti-infective
GENERAL USES:
Bacterial infections
DOSAGE FORMS:
Tablets: 200 mg

CEFEPIME
SEF e pim
TRADE NAME(S):
Maxipime
THERAPEUTIC CLASS:
Anti-infective

GENERAL USES:
Bacterial infections
DOSAGE FORMS:
Injection: 500 mg, 1 g, 2 g

CEFIXIME
sef IKS eem
TRADE NAME(S):
Suprax
THERAPEUTIC CLASS:
Anti-infective
GENERAL USES:
Bacterial infections
DOSAGE FORMS:
Tablets: 200 mg, 400 mg;
Suspension: 100 mg/
5 mL

CEFMETAZOLE
sef MET ah zole
TRADE NAME(S):
Zefazone
THERAPEUTIC CLASS:
Anti-infective
GENERAL USES:
Bacterial infections
DOSAGE FORMS:
Injection: 1 g, 2 g

CEFONICID
se FON i sid
TRADE NAME(S):
Monocid
THERAPEUTIC CLASS:
Anti-infective
GENERAL USES:
Bacterial infections

DOSAGE FORMS:
Injection: 1 g, 10 g

CEFOPERAZONE
sef oh PER a zone
TRADE NAME(S):
Cefobid
THERAPEUTIC CLASS:
Anti-infective
GENERAL USES:
Bacterial infections
DOSAGE FORMS:
Injection: 1 g, 2 g, 10 g

CEFOTAXIME SODIUM
sef oh TAKS eem
TRADE NAME(S):
Claforan
THERAPEUTIC CLASS:
Anti-infective
GENERAL USES:
Bacterial infections
DOSAGE FORMS:
Injection: 500 mg, 1 g,
2 g, 10 g

CEFOXITIN SODIUM
se FOKS i tin
TRADE NAME(S):
Mefoxin
THERAPEUTIC CLASS:
Anti-infective
GENERAL USES:
Bacterial infections
DOSAGE FORMS:
Injection: 1 g, 2 g, 10 g

CEFPODOXIME
sef pode OKS eem

TRADE NAME(S):
Vantin

THERAPEUTIC CLASS:
Anti-infective

GENERAL USES:
Bacterial infections

DOSAGE FORMS:
Tablets: 100 mg, 200 mg;
Suspension: 50 mg/5 mL,
100 mg/5 mL

CEFPROZIL
sef PROE zil

TRADE NAME(S):
Cefzil

THERAPEUTIC CLASS:
Anti-infective

GENERAL USES:
Bacterial infections

DOSAGE FORMS:
Capsules: 250 mg,
500 mg; Suspension:
125 mg/5 mL, 250 mg/
5 mL

CEFTAZIDIME
SEF tay zi deem

TRADE NAME(S):
Fortaz, Ceptaz, Tazidime

THERAPEUTIC CLASS:
Anti-infective

GENERAL USES:
Bacterial infections

DOSAGE FORMS:
Injection: 500 mg, 1 g,
2 g, 6 g, 10 g

CEFTIBUTEN
sef TYE byoo ten

TRADE NAME(S):
Cedax

THERAPEUTIC CLASS:
Anti-infective

GENERAL USES:
Bacterial infections

DOSAGE FORMS:
Capsules: 400 mg;
Suspension: 90 mg/5 mL,
180 mg/5 mL

CEFTIZOXIME SODIUM
sef ti ZOKS eem

TRADE NAME(S):
Cefizox

THERAPEUTIC CLASS:
Anti-infective

GENERAL USES:
Bacterial infections

DOSAGE FORMS:
Injection: 500 mg, 1 g,
2 g, 10 g

CEFTRIAXONE SODIUM
sef trye AKS one

TRADE NAME(S):
Rocephin

THERAPEUTIC CLASS:
Anti-infective

GENERAL USES:
Bacterial infections

DOSAGE FORMS:
Injection: 250 mg,
500 mg, 1 g, 2 g, 10 g

CEFUROXIME AXETIL
se fyoor OKS eem
AKS e til
TRADE NAME(S):
Ceftin
THERAPEUTIC CLASS:
Anti-infective
GENERAL USES:
Bacterial infections
DOSAGE FORMS:
Tablets: 125 mg, 250 mg,
500 mg; Suspension:
125 mg/5 mL, 250 mg/
5 mL

CEFUROXIME SODIUM
se fyoor OKS eem
TRADE NAME(S):
Zinacef
THERAPEUTIC CLASS:
Anti-infective
GENERAL USES:
Bacterial infections
DOSAGE FORMS:
Injection: 750 mg, 1.5 mg,
7.5 g

CELECOXIB
se le KOKS ib
TRADE NAME(S):
Celebrex
THERAPEUTIC CLASS:
Anti-inflammatory/
analgesic
GENERAL USES:
Osteoarthritis, rheumatoid
arthritis, dysmenorrhea,

FAP, acute pain
DOSAGE FORMS:
Capsules: 100 mg,
200 mg

CEPHALEXIN
sef a LEKS in
TRADE NAME(S):
Keflex, Biocef
THERAPEUTIC CLASS:
Anti-infective
GENERAL USES:
Bacterial infections
DOSAGE FORMS:
Capsules: 250 mg,
333 mg, 500 mg, 750 mg;
Tablets: 250 mg, 500 mg;
Suspension: 125 mg/
5 mL, 250 mg/5 mL

CEPHALEXIN HCL
sef a LEKS in
TRADE NAME(S):
Keftab
THERAPEUTIC CLASS:
Anti-infective
GENERAL USES:
Bacterial infections
DOSAGE FORMS:
Tablets: 500 mg

CEPHRADINE
SEF ra deen
TRADE NAME(S):
Velosef
THERAPEUTIC CLASS:
Anti-infective

GENERAL USES:
  Bacterial infections
DOSAGE FORMS:
  Capsules: 250 mg,
  500 mg; Suspension:
  125 mg/5 mL, 250 mg/
  5 mL; Injection: 250 mg,
  500 mg, 1 g, 2 g

CERTOLIZUMAB PEGOL
SER toe LIZ oo mab peg OL
TRADE NAME(S):
  Cimzia
THERAPEUTIC CLASS:
  Tumor necrosis factor
GENERAL USES:
  Crohn's disease
DOSAGE FORMS:
  Injection: 200 mg

CETIRIZINE
se TI ra zeen
TRADE NAME(S):
  Zyrtec
THERAPEUTIC CLASS:
  Antihistamine
GENERAL USES:
  Allergic rhinitis/hives
DOSAGE FORMS:
  Tablets and Chewable
  tablets: 5 mg, 10 mg;
  Syrup: 5 mg/5 mL

CETIRIZINE/ PSEUDOEPHEDRINE
se TI ra zeen/soo doe e FED
rin

TRADE NAME(S):
  Zyrtec-D
THERAPEUTIC CLASS:
  Antihistamine/
  decongestant
GENERAL USES:
  Allergies
DOSAGE FORMS:
  Extended-release tablets:
  5 mg/120 mg

CETRORELIX ACETATE
set roe REL iks
TRADE NAME(S):
  Cetrotide
THERAPEUTIC CLASS:
  Hormone antagonist
GENERAL USES:
  Prevention of LH surges
DOSAGE FORMS:
  Injection: 0.25 mg, 3 mg

CETUXIMAB
se TUK see mab
TRADE NAME(S):
  Erbitux
THERAPEUTIC CLASS:
  Antineoplastic
GENERAL USES:
  Various cancers
DOSAGE FORMS:
  Injection: 100 mg

CEVIMELINE
se vi ME leen
TRADE NAME(S):
  Evoxac

THERAPEUTIC CLASS:
Saliva stimulant
GENERAL USES:
Dry mouth in Sjögren's
syndrome
DOSAGE FORMS:
Capsules: 30 mg

CHLORAL HYDRATE
KLOR al HYE drate
TRADE NAME(S):
Aquachloral
Supprettes
THERAPEUTIC CLASS:
Sedative/hypnotic
GENERAL USES:
Pre-op sedation
DOSAGE FORMS:
Capsules: 500 mg; Syrup:
250 mg/5 mL, 500 mg/
5 mL

CHLORAMPHENICOL (OCULAR)
klor am FEN i kole
TRADE NAME(S):
AK-Chlor, Chloroptic,
Ocuchlor
THERAPEUTIC CLASS:
Ocular agent (anti-
infective)
GENERAL USES:
Ocular infections
DOSAGE FORMS:
Ophthalmic solution:
5 mg/mL; Ophthalmic
ointment: 10 mg/g

CHLORAMPHENICOL (ORAL)
klor am FEN i kole
TRADE NAME(S):
Chloromycetin
THERAPEUTIC CLASS:
Anti-infective
GENERAL USES:
Bacterial infections
DOSAGE FORMS:
Capsules: 250 mg;
Injection: 1 g

CHLORDIAZEPOXIDE
klor dye az e POKS ide
TRADE NAME(S):
Librium, Mitran, Libritabs
THERAPEUTIC CLASS:
Antianxiety agent,
anticonvulsant
GENERAL USES:
Anxiety, alcohol
withdrawal, seizures
DOSAGE FORMS:
Capsules: 5 mg, 10 mg,
25 mg; Tablets: 10 mg,
25 mg; Injection: 100 mg

CHLORDIAZEPOXIDE/ AMITRIPTYLINE
klor dye az e POKS ide/a
mee TRIP ti leen
TRADE NAME(S):
Limbitrol DS
THERAPEUTIC CLASS:
Sedative/antidepressant
GENERAL USES:
Depression/anxiety

DOSAGE FORMS:
Tablets: 5 mg/12.5 mg,
10 mg/25 mg

CHLOROQUINE PHOSPHATE
KLOR oh kwin
TRADE NAME(S):
Aralen
THERAPEUTIC CLASS:
Antimalarial
GENERAL USES:
Malaria treatment
and prevention,
intestinal
amebiasis
DOSAGE FORMS:
Tablets: 250 mg, 500 mg

CHLOROTHIAZIDE
klor oh THYE a zide
TRADE NAME(S):
Diuril
THERAPEUTIC CLASS:
Diuretic
GENERAL USES:
CHF-related edema,
hypertension
DOSAGE FORMS:
Tablets: 250 mg, 500 mg;
Suspension: 250 mg/
5 mL

CHLORPROMAZINE
klor PROE ma zeen
TRADE NAME(S):
Thorazine

THERAPEUTIC CLASS:
Antipsychotic
GENERAL USES:
Psychotic/behavioral
disorders, porphyria,
emesis
DOSAGE FORMS:
Tablets: 10 mg, 25 mg,
50 mg, 100 mg, 200 mg;
Sustained-release
capsules: 30 mg, 75 mg,
150 mg, 200 mg, 300 mg;
Syrup: 10 mg/5 mL;
Concentrated solution:
30 mg/mL, 100 mg/mL;
Injection: 25 mg, 50 mg

CHLORPROPAMIDE
klor PROE pa mide
TRADE NAME(S):
Diabinese
THERAPEUTIC CLASS:
Antidiabetic
GENERAL USES:
Diabetes (type 2)
DOSAGE FORMS:
Tablets: 100 mg, 250 mg

CHLORTHALIDONE
klor THAL i done
TRADE NAME(S):
Thalitone, Hygroton
THERAPEUTIC CLASS:
Diuretic
GENERAL USES:
CHF-related edema,
hypertension

DOSAGE FORMS:
Tablets: 15 mg, 25 mg,
50 mg, 100 mg

CHLORZOXAZONE
klor ZOKS a zone
TRADE NAME(S):
Paraflex, Parafon Forte
DSC, Remular
THERAPEUTIC CLASS:
Skeletal muscle relaxant
GENERAL USES:
Musculoskeletal
conditions
DOSAGE FORMS:
Tablets and Capsules:
250 mg, 500 mg

CICLESONIDE
sye KLE soh nide
TRADE NAME(S):
Omnaris
THERAPEUTIC CLASS:
Corticosteroid
GENERAL USES:
Seasonal and perennial
allergies
DOSAGE FORMS:
Nasal spray: 50 mcg

CICLOPIROX
sye kloe PEER oks
TRADE NAME(S):
Loprox, Penlac
THERAPEUTIC CLASS:
Antifungal (topical)
GENERAL USES:
Athlete's foot, jock itch,
ringworm, nail infections
(topical nail
preparation)
DOSAGE FORMS:
Cream and Lotion: 1%;
Nail lacquer: 8%

CILOSTAZOL
sil OH sta zol
TRADE NAME(S):
Pletal
THERAPEUTIC CLASS:
Antiplatelet agent
GENERAL USES:
Intermittent
claudication
DOSAGE FORMS:
Tablets: 50 mg, 100 mg

CIMETIDINE
sye MET i deen
TRADE NAME(S):
Tagamet, Tagamet HB
THERAPEUTIC CLASS:
Gastric acid secretion
inhibitor
GENERAL USES:
Duodenal ulcer, GERD,
heartburn (OTC)
DOSAGE FORMS:
Tablets: 100 mg, 200 mg,
300 mg, 400 mg, 800 mg;
Solution: 300 mg/5 mL;
Injection: 300 mg, 600 mg

CINACALCET
sin a KAL set
TRADE NAME(S):
Sensipar

Therapeutic Class:
Hyperparathyroid agent
General Uses:
Secondary hyperparathyroidism, hypercalcemia in parathyroid cancer
Dosage Forms:
Tablets: 30 mg, 60 mg, 90 mg

CINOXACIN
sin OKS a sin
Trade Name(s):
Cinobac
Therapeutic Class:
Anti-infective
General Uses:
Bacterial infections
Dosage Forms:
Capsules: 250 mg, 500 mg

CIPROFLOXACIN
sip roe FLOKS a sin
Trade Name(s):
Cipro, Cipro XR, Proquin XR
Therapeutic Class:
Anti-infective
General Uses:
Bacterial infections
Dosage Forms:
Tablets: 100 mg, 250 mg, 500 mg, 750 mg; Extended-release tablets: 500 mg, 1000 mg;

Suspension: 250 mg/5 mL, 500 mg/5 mL; Injection: 200 mg, 400 mg

CIPROFLOXACIN (OCULAR)
sip roe FLOKS a sin
Trade Name(s):
Ciloxan
Therapeutic Class:
Ocular agent (anti-infective)
General Uses:
Ocular infections
Dosage Forms:
Ophthalmic solution and Ointment: 0.3%

CIPROFLOXACIN/ DEXAMETHASONE (OTIC)
sip roe FLOKS a sin/deks a METH a sone
Trade Name(s):
Ciprodex
Therapeutic Class:
Otic agent (anti-infective/anti-inflammatory)
General Uses:
Acute otitis media
Dosage Forms:
Otic suspension: 0.3%/0.1%

CIPROFLOXACIN/ HYDROCORTISONE (OTIC)
sip roe FLOKS a sin/ hye droe KOR ti sone

TRADE NAME(S):
Cipro HC

THERAPEUTIC CLASS:
Otic agent (anti-infective/ anti-inflammatory)

GENERAL USES:
Acute otitis media

DOSAGE FORMS:
Otic suspension: 2 mg/ 10 mg per mL

CISPLATIN
SIS pla tin

TRADE NAME(S):
Platinol-AQ

THERAPEUTIC CLASS:
Antineoplastic

GENERAL USES:
Cancer of the bladder, testes, ovaries

DOSAGE FORMS:
Injection: 50 mg, 100 mg, 200 mg

CITALOPRAM
sye TAL oh pram

TRADE NAME(S):
Celexa

THERAPEUTIC CLASS:
Antidepressant

GENERAL USES:
Depression

DOSAGE FORMS:
Tablets: 20 mg, 40 mg; Solution: 10 mg/ 5 mL

CLARITHROMYCIN
kla RITH roe mye sin

TRADE NAME(S):
Biaxin, Biaxin XL

THERAPEUTIC CLASS:
Anti-infective

GENERAL USES:
Bacterial infections

DOSAGE FORMS:
Tablets: 250 mg; Tablets and Extended-release tablets: 500 mg; Suspension: 125 mg/ 5 mL, 250 mg/5 mL

CLEVIDIPINE BUTYRATE
kle VID i peen

TRADE NAME(S):
Cleviprex

THERAPEUTIC CLASS:
Antihypertensive

GENERAL USES:
Hypertension

DOSAGE FORMS:
Injection: 25 mg, 50 mg

CLINDAMYCIN
klin da MYE sin

TRADE NAME(S):
Cleocin

Therapeutic Class:
Anti-infective
General Uses:
Bacterial infections
Dosage Forms:
Capsules: 75 mg, 150 mg,
300 mg; Solution: 75 mg/
5 mL; Injection: 300 mg,
600 mg, 900 mg

CLINDAMYCIN (TOPICAL)
klin da MYE sin
Trade Name(s):
Cleocin T, Clinda-Derm
Therapeutic Class:
Anti-infective (topical)
General Uses:
Acne
Dosage Forms:
Gel, Lotion, and Topical
solution: 10 mg/mL

CLINDAMYCIN (VAGINAL)
klin da MYE sin
Trade Name(s):
Cleocin, Clindesse
Therapeutic Class:
Vaginal anti-infective
General Uses:
Vaginal bacterial
infections
Dosage Forms:
Cream: 2%

CLOBETASOL
kloe BAY ta sol

Trade Name(s):
Temovate, Olux-E
Therapeutic Class:
Corticosteroid (topical)
General Uses:
Various skin conditions
Dosage Forms:
Ointment, Cream, Foam,
Gel, Lotion, Solution,
Shampoo, and Topical
spray: 0.05%

CLOFARABINE
kloe FAR a been
Trade Name(s):
Clolar
Therapeutic Class:
Antineoplastic
General Uses:
Pediatric cancer (ALL)
Dosage Forms:
Injection: 20 mg

CLOMIPRAMINE
kloe MI pra meen
Trade Name(s):
Anafranil
Therapeutic Class:
Antidepressant
General Uses:
OCD
Dosage Forms:
Capsules: 25 mg, 50 mg,
75 mg

CLONAZEPAM
kloe NA ze pam

TRADE NAME(S):
Klonopin

THERAPEUTIC CLASS:
Anticonvulsant

GENERAL USES:
Seizures

DOSAGE FORMS:
Tablets: 0.5 mg, 1 mg,
2 mg

CLONIDINE
KLON i deen

TRADE NAME(S):
Catapres, Catapres-TTS

THERAPEUTIC CLASS:
Antihypertensive

GENERAL USES:
Hypertension

DOSAGE FORMS:
Tablets: 0.1 mg, 0.2 mg,
0.3 mg; Transdermal
patch (content): 2.5 mg,
5 mg, 7.5 mg

CLONIDINE/
CHLORTHALIDONE
KLON i deen/klor THAL i done

TRADE NAME(S):
Combipres

THERAPEUTIC CLASS:
Antihypertensive/diuretic

GENERAL USES:
Hypertension

DOSAGE FORMS:
Tablets: 0.1 mg/15 mg,
0.2 mg/15 mg, 0.3 mg/
15 mg

CLOPIDOGREL
kloh PID oh grel

TRADE NAME(S):
Plavix

THERAPEUTIC CLASS:
Antiplatelet agent

GENERAL USES:
Reduce stroke, MI risk,
acute coronary syndrome

DOSAGE FORMS:
Tablets: 75 mg

CLORAZEPATE
klor AZ e pate

TRADE NAME(S):
Tranxene, Gen-Xene

THERAPEUTIC CLASS:
Antianxiety agent,
anticonvulsant

GENERAL USES:
Anxiety, panic disorder,
seizures

DOSAGE FORMS:
Capsules or Tablets:
3.75 mg, 7.5 mg, 15 mg;
Single-dose tablets:
11.25 mg, 22.5 mg

CLOTRIMAZOLE (ORAL)
kloe TRIM a zole

TRADE NAME(S):
Mycelex

THERAPEUTIC CLASS:
Antifungal

GENERAL USES:
Oral fungal infection
(candidiasis)

DOSAGE FORMS:
Troches: 10 mg

CLOTRIMAZOLE (TOPICAL)
kloe TRIM a zole
TRADE NAME(S):
Lotrimin, Mycelex
THERAPEUTIC CLASS:
Antifungal (topical)
GENERAL USES:
Athlete's foot, jock itch, ringworm, tinea versicolor, candidiasis
DOSAGE FORMS:
Cream, Solution, and Lotion: 1%

CLOXACILLIN
kloks a SIL in
TRADE NAME(S):
Cloxapen
THERAPEUTIC CLASS:
Anti-infective
GENERAL USES:
Bacterial infections
DOSAGE FORMS:
Capsules: 250 mg, 500 mg; Solution: 125 mg/5 mL

CLOZAPINE
KLOE za peen
TRADE NAME(S):
Clozaril
THERAPEUTIC CLASS:
Antipsychotic
GENERAL USES:
Psychotic

disorders
DOSAGE FORMS:
Tablets: 25 mg, 100 mg, 200 mg; Orally disintegrating tablets: 25 mg, 100 mg

CODEINE SULFATE
KOE deen
TRADE NAME(S):
Codeine
THERAPEUTIC CLASS:
Analgesic (narcotic)
GENERAL USES:
Pain, cough
DOSAGE FORMS:
Tablets: 15 mg, 30 mg, 60 mg; Soluble tablets: 30 mg, 60 mg

COLCHICINE
KOL chi seen
TRADE NAME(S):
Colchicine
THERAPEUTIC CLASS:
Gout agent
GENERAL USES:
Gout
DOSAGE FORMS:
Tablets: 0.5 mg, 0.6 mg

COLESEVELAM
koh le SEV a lam
TRADE NAME(S):
Welchol
THERAPEUTIC CLASS:
Antilipemic

GENERAL USES:
Hyperlipidemia
DOSAGE FORMS:
Tablets: 625 mg

CONIVAPTAN
koe NYE vap tan
TRADE NAME(S):
Vaprisol
THERAPEUTIC CLASS:
Vasopressin receptor antagonist
GENERAL USES:
Euvolemic hyponatremia
DOSAGE FORMS:
Injection: 20 mg

CROMOLYN (INHALED)
KROE moe lin
TRADE NAME(S):
Intal
THERAPEUTIC CLASS:
Respiratory inhalant
GENERAL USES:
Asthma, bronchospasm
DOSAGE FORMS:
Aerosol spray: 800 mcg/ spray; Nebulizer solution: 20 mg/2 mL

CROMOLYN (OCULAR)
KROE moe lin
TRADE NAME(S):
Crolom
THERAPEUTIC CLASS:
Ocular agent
GENERAL USES:
Conjunctivitis

DOSAGE FORMS:
Ophthalmic solution: 4%

CROMOLYN (ORAL)
KROE moe lin
TRADE NAME(S):
Gastrocrom
THERAPEUTIC CLASS:
Mast cell stabilizer
GENERAL USES:
Mastocytosis
DOSAGE FORMS:
Oral concentrate: 100 mg/ 5 mL

CROTAMITON
kroe TAM i ton
TRADE NAME(S):
Eurax
THERAPEUTIC CLASS:
Scabicide (topical)
GENERAL USES:
Scabies, pruritus
DOSAGE FORMS:
Cream and Lotion: 10%

CYANOCOBALAMIN
sye an oh koe BAL a min
TRADE NAME(S):
Nascobal, Vitamin B-12
THERAPEUTIC CLASS:
Vitamin
GENERAL USES:
Vitamin B12 deficiency
DOSAGE FORMS:
Nasal gel: 500 mcg/ 0.1 mL; Nasal spray:

500 mcg/0.1 mL;
Injection: 1000 mcg/mL;
Tablets: 50 mcg, 100 mcg,
250 mcg, 500 mcg,
1000 mcg, 5000 mcg;
Extended-release tablets:
1500 mcg; Sublingual
tablets: 2500 mcg;
Lozenges: 100 mcg,
250 mcg, 500 mcg

CYCLOBENZAPRINE
sye kloe BEN za preen
TRADE NAME(S):
Flexeril
THERAPEUTIC CLASS:
Skeletal muscle
relaxant
GENERAL USES:
Musculoskeletal
conditions
DOSAGE FORMS:
Tablets: 5 mg, 7.5 mg,
10 mg

CYCLOPHOSPHAMIDE
sye kloe FOS fa mide
TRADE NAME(S):
Cytoxan
THERAPEUTIC CLASS:
Antineoplastic
GENERAL USES:
Various lymphomas and
leukemias
DOSAGE FORMS:
Tablets: 25 mg, 50 mg;
Injection: 100 mg,
200 mg, 500 mg, 1 g, 2 g

CYCLOSERINE
sye kloe SER een
TRADE NAME(S):
Seromycin
THERAPEUTIC CLASS:
Antituberculosis
agent
GENERAL USES:
Tuberculosis
DOSAGE FORMS:
Capsules: 250 mg

CYCLOSPORINE
SYE kloe spor een
TRADE NAME(S):
Sandimmune, Neoral,
SangCya
THERAPEUTIC CLASS:
Immunosuppressant
GENERAL USES:
Rheumatoid arthritis,
psoriasis, prevent organ
rejection
DOSAGE FORMS:
Capsules: 25 mg, 50 mg,
100 mg; Solution:
100 mg/mL; Injection:
250 mg

CYCLOSPORINE
(OCULAR)
SYE kloe spor een
TRADE NAME(S):
Restasis
THERAPEUTIC CLASS:
Ocular agent (anti-
inflammatory)

GENERAL USES:
Increase tear production
DOSAGE FORMS:
Ophthalmic emulsion:
0.05%

CYPROHEPTADINE
si proe HEP ta deen
TRADE NAME(S):
Periactin
THERAPEUTIC CLASS:
Antihistamine
GENERAL USES:
Allergies
DOSAGE FORMS:
Tablets: 4 mg; Syrup:
2 mg/5 mL

DALTEPARIN SODIUM
dal TE pa rin
TRADE NAME(S):
Fragmin
THERAPEUTIC CLASS:
Anticoagulant (LMWH)
GENERAL USES:
Prevention of blood clots
DOSAGE FORMS:
Injection:
2500 international units,
5000 international units,
95,000 international units

DANAPAROID SODIUM
da NAP a roid
TRADE NAME(S):
Orgaran

THERAPEUTIC CLASS:
Anticoagulant
GENERAL USES:
Prevention of blood clots
DOSAGE FORMS:
Injection: 750 anti-Xa
units

DANTROLENE
DAN troe leen
TRADE NAME(S):
Dantrium
THERAPEUTIC CLASS:
Skeletal muscle relaxant
GENERAL USES:
Spasticity
DOSAGE FORMS:
Capsules: 25 mg, 50 mg,
100 mg; Injection: 20 mg

DAPSONE
DAP sone
TRADE NAME(S):
Aczone
THERAPEUTIC CLASS:
Dermatologic agent
GENERAL USES:
Acne vulgaris
DOSAGE FORMS:
Gel: 5%

DAPTOMYCIN
DAP toe mye sin
TRADE NAME(S):
Cubicin
THERAPEUTIC CLASS:
Anti-infective

GENERAL USES:
Bacterial infections
DOSAGE FORMS:
Injection: 250 mg, 500 mg

DARBEPOETIN ALFA
dar be POE e tin AL fa
TRADE NAME(S):
Aranesp
THERAPEUTIC CLASS:
Hematological agent
GENERAL USES:
Anemia
DOSAGE FORMS:
Injection: 0.025 mg,
0.04 mg, 0.06 mg, 0.1 mg,
0.15 mg, 0.2 mg, 0.3 mg,
0.5 mg

**DARIFENACIN
HYDROBROMIDE**
dar i FEN a sin
TRADE NAME(S):
Enablex
THERAPEUTIC CLASS:
Anticholinergic
GENERAL USES:
Overactive bladder
DOSAGE FORMS:
Extended-release tablets:
7.5 mg, 15 mg

DARUNAVIR
da ROO na veer
TRADE NAME(S):
Prezista
THERAPEUTIC CLASS:
Antiviral

GENERAL USES:
HIV infection
DOSAGE FORMS:
Tablets: 300 mg

DASATINIB
da SA ti nib
TRADE NAME(S):
Sprycel
THERAPEUTIC CLASS:
Antineoplastic
GENERAL USES:
Myeloid leukemia
DOSAGE FORMS:
Tablets: 20 mg, 50 mg,
70 mg

DECITABINE
de SYE ta been
TRADE NAME(S):
Dacogen
THERAPEUTIC CLASS:
Antineoplastic
GENERAL USES:
Myelodysplastic disease
DOSAGE FORMS:
Injection: 50 mg

DEFERASIROX
de FER a sir oks
TRADE NAME(S):
Exjade
THERAPEUTIC CLASS:
Chelating agent
GENERAL USES:
Chronic iron overload due
to blood transfusions

DOSAGE FORMS:
Tablets: 125 mg, 250 mg, 500 mg

DELAVIRDINE
de la VIR deen
TRADE NAME(S):
Rescriptor
THERAPEUTIC CLASS:
Antiviral
GENERAL USES:
HIV infection
DOSAGE FORMS:
Tablets: 100 mg, 200 mg

DEMECARIUM
dem e KARE ee um
TRADE NAME(S):
Humorsol
THERAPEUTIC CLASS:
Ocular agent
GENERAL USES:
Glaucoma
DOSAGE FORMS:
Ophthalmic solution: 0.125%, 0.25%

DEMECLOCYCLINE
dem e kloe SYE kleen
TRADE NAME(S):
Declomycin
THERAPEUTIC CLASS:
Anti-infective
GENERAL USES:
Bacterial infections
DOSAGE FORMS:
Tablets: 150 mg, 300 mg

DESIPRAMINE
des IP ra meen
TRADE NAME(S):
Norpramin
THERAPEUTIC CLASS:
Antidepressant
GENERAL USES:
Depression
DOSAGE FORMS:
Tablets: 10 mg, 25 mg, 50 mg, 75 mg, 100 mg, 150 mg

DESLORATADINE
des lor AT a deen
TRADE NAME(S):
Clarinex, Clarinex Redi-tabs
THERAPEUTIC CLASS:
Antihistamine
GENERAL USES:
Allergic rhinitis, chronic urticaria
DOSAGE FORMS:
Tablets: 5 mg; Orally disintegrating tablets: 2.5 mg, 5 mg; Syrup: 0.5 mg/mL

DESLORATADINE/ PSEUDOEPHEDRINE
des lor AT a deen/soo doe e FED rin
TRADE NAME(S):
Clarinex-D 12 hour, Clarinex-D 24 hour
THERAPEUTIC CLASS:
Antihistamine/

Decongestant
GENERAL USES:
Seasonal allergic rhinitis
DOSAGE FORMS:
Tablets (various release):
2.5 mg/120 mg, 5 mg/
240 mg

DESONIDE
DES oh nide
TRADE NAME(S):
DesOwen, Tridesilon,
Verdeso
THERAPEUTIC CLASS:
Corticosteroid (topical)
GENERAL USES:
Various skin conditions
DOSAGE FORMS:
Ointment, Cream, Foam,
and Lotion: 0.05%

DESVENLAFAXINE
des VEN la FAX een
TRADE NAME(S):
Pristiq
THERAPEUTIC CLASS:
Antidepressant
GENERAL USES:
Depression
DOSAGE FORMS:
Tablets: 50 mg, 100 mg

DEXAMETHASONE
(OCULAR)
deks a METH a sone
TRADE NAME(S):
AK-Dex, Maxidex

THERAPEUTIC CLASS:
Ocular agent (steroid)
GENERAL USES:
Ocular inflammation
DOSAGE FORMS:
Ophthalmic solution,
Suspension, Ointment:
0.1%

DEXAMETHASONE
(ORAL)
deks a METH a sone
TRADE NAME(S):
Decadron, Dexone,
Hexadrol
THERAPEUTIC CLASS:
Glucocorticoid
GENERAL USES:
Endocrine, skin, blood
disorders
DOSAGE FORMS:
Tablets: 0.25 mg, 0.5 mg,
0.75 mg, 1 mg, 1.5 mg,
2 mg, 4 mg, 6 mg; Elixir
and Solution: 0.5 mg/
5 mL; Concentrated
solution: 1 mg/1 mL

DEXAMETHASONE
ACETATE
deks a METH a sone
TRADE NAME(S):
Dalalone LA, Decadron LA
THERAPEUTIC CLASS:
Glucocorticoid
GENERAL USES:
Endocrine, skin, blood

disorders

DOSAGE FORMS:
Injection: 8 mg, 16 mg,
40 mg, 80 mg

DEXAMETHASONE SODIUM PHOSPHATE
deks a METH a sone

TRADE NAME(S):
Dalalone, Decadron
Phosphate, Dexasone

THERAPEUTIC CLASS:
Glucocorticoid

GENERAL USES:
Endocrine, skin, blood
disorders

DOSAGE FORMS:
Injection: 4 mg, 10 mg,
20 mg, 40 mg, 100 mg,
120 mg, 240 mg

DEXMETHYLPHENIDATE
deks meth il FEN i date

TRADE NAME(S):
Focalin, Focalin XR

THERAPEUTIC CLASS:
CNS stimulant

GENERAL USES:
ADHD

DOSAGE FORMS:
Tablets: 2.5 mg, 5 mg,
10 mg; Extended-release
capsules: 5 mg, 10 mg,
20 mg

DEXTROAMPHETAMINE SULFATE
deks troe am FET a meen

TRADE NAME(S):
Dexedrine

THERAPEUTIC CLASS:
Amphetamine

GENERAL USES:
Obesity

DOSAGE FORMS:
Tablets: 5 mg, 10 mg;
Sustained-release
capsules: 5 mg, 10 mg,
15 mg; Elixir:
5 mg/5 mL

DEXTROAMPHETAMINE/ AMPHETAMINE
deks troe am FET a meen/am
FET a meen

TRADE NAME(S):
Adderall, Adderall XR

THERAPEUTIC CLASS:
Amphetamine

GENERAL USES:
ADHD

DOSAGE FORMS:
Tablets: 5 mg, 10 mg,
20 mg, 30 mg; Extended-
release capsules: 10 mg,
20 mg, 30 mg

DIAZEPAM
dye AZ e pam

TRADE NAME(S):
Valium

THERAPEUTIC CLASS:
Antianxiety agent,
anticonvulsant, muscle
relaxant

GENERAL USES:
Anxiety, alcohol
withdrawal, seizures,
muscle relaxant
DOSAGE FORMS:
Tablets: 2 mg, 5 mg,
10 mg; Solution: 5 mg/
5 mL, 5 mg/mL; Injection:
10 mg, 50 mg

DICLOFENAC (OCULAR)
dye KLOE fen ak
TRADE NAME(S):
Voltaren
THERAPEUTIC CLASS:
Ocular agent
GENERAL USES:
Postoperative ocular
inflammation
DOSAGE FORMS:
Ophthalmic solution: 0.1%

DICLOFENAC (ORAL)
dye KLOE fen ak
TRADE NAME(S):
Cataflam, Voltaren,
Voltaren-XR
THERAPEUTIC CLASS:
Anti-inflammatory/
analgesic
GENERAL USES:
Osteoarthritis, rheumatoid
arthritis, pain
DOSAGE FORMS:
Tablets and Delayed-
release tablets: 25 mg,
50 mg, 75 mg; Extended-
release tablets: 100 mg

DICLOFENAC EPOLAMINE (TRANSDERMAL)
dye KLOE fen ak
TRADE NAME(S):
Flector
THERAPEUTIC CLASS:
Anti-inflammatory/
analgesic
GENERAL USES:
Acute pain
DOSAGE FORMS:
Patch: 180 mg

DICLOFENAC/ MISOPROSTOL
dye KLOE fen ak/mye soe
PROST ole
TRADE NAME(S):
Arthrotec
THERAPEUTIC CLASS:
Analgesic/GI protectant
GENERAL USES:
Arthritis
DOSAGE FORMS:
Tablets: 50 mg/200 mcg,
75 mg/200 mcg

DICLOXACILLIN
dye kloks a SIL in
TRADE NAME(S):
Dynapen, Dycill, Pathocil
THERAPEUTIC CLASS:
Anti-infective
GENERAL USES:
Bacterial infections

DOSAGE FORMS:
Capsules: 125 mg,
250 mg, 500 mg;
Suspension: 62.5 mg/
5 mL

DICYCLOMINE
dye SYE kloe meen
TRADE NAME(S):
Bentyl, Byclomine, Di-Spaz
THERAPEUTIC CLASS:
GI antispasmodic
GENERAL USES:
Irritable bowel syndrome
DOSAGE FORMS:
Capsules: 10 mg, 20 mg;
Tablets: 20 mg; Syrup:
10 mg/5 mL

DIDANOSINE (ddl)
dye DAN oh seen
TRADE NAME(S):
Videx, Videx EC
THERAPEUTIC CLASS:
Antiviral
GENERAL USES:
HIV infection
DOSAGE FORMS:
Chewable tablets: 25 mg,
50 mg, 100 mg, 150 mg,
200 mg; Powder: 100 mg,
167 mg, 250 mg, 375 mg,
2 g, 4 g; Delayed-release
capsules: 125 mg,
200 mg, 250 mg,
400 mg

DIFLUNISAL
dye FLOO ni sal
TRADE NAME(S):
Dolobid
THERAPEUTIC CLASS:
Anti-inflammatory/
analgesic
GENERAL USES:
Pain, osteoarthritis,
rheumatoid arthritis
DOSAGE FORMS:
Tablets: 250 mg, 500 mg

DIFLUPREDNATE (OCULAR)
DYE floo PRED nate
TRADE NAME(S):
Durezol
THERAPEUTIC CLASS:
Corticosteroid (ocular)
GENERAL USES:
Surgically induced ocular
inflammation and pain
DOSAGE FORMS:
Ophthalmic solution:
0.05%

DIGOXIN
di JOKS in
TRADE NAME(S):
Lanoxicaps, Lanoxin,
Digitek
THERAPEUTIC CLASS:
Cardiac agent
GENERAL USES:
CHF, atrial fibrillation
DOSAGE FORMS:

Capsules: 0.05 mg,
0.1 mg, 0.2 mg; Tablets:
0.125 mg, 0.25 mg; Elixir:
0.05 mg/mL; Injection:
0.1 mg, 0.25 mg, 0.5 mg

DIHYDROERGOTAMINE
dye hye droe er GOT a meen
TRADE NAME(S):
Migranal
THERAPEUTIC CLASS:
Anti-migraine agent
GENERAL USES:
Migraines
DOSAGE FORMS:
Nasal spray: 4 mg/mL

DILTIAZEM
dil TYE a zem
TRADE NAME(S):
Cardizem CD,
Cardizem LA,
Dilacor XR, Tiazac,
Taztia XT
THERAPEUTIC CLASS:
Antihypertensive,
antianginal
GENERAL USES:
Hypertension, angina
DOSAGE FORMS:
Tablets: 30 mg, 60 mg,
90 mg, 120 mg;
Extended-release
capsules and Tablets:
120 mg, 180 mg, 240 mg,
300 mg, 360 mg, 420 mg;
Injection: 25 mg, 50 mg,
125 mg

DILTIAZEM/ENALAPRIL
dil TYE a zem/e NAL a pril
TRADE NAME(S):
Teczem
THERAPEUTIC CLASS:
Antihypertensive
GENERAL USES:
Hypertension
DOSAGE FORMS:
Extended-release tablets:
180 mg/5 mg

DIMENHYDRINATE
dye men HYE drih nate
TRADE NAME(S):
Hydrate, Dramanate
THERAPEUTIC CLASS:
Antiemetic/antivertigo
agent
GENERAL USES:
Motion sickness
DOSAGE FORMS:
Tablets: 50 mg

DIPHENHYDRAMINE
dye fen HYE dra meen
TRADE NAME(S):
Benadryl, Tusstat,
Hyrexin-50
THERAPEUTIC CLASS:
Antihistamine, antiemetic
GENERAL USES:
Pruritus, allergies, sleep
aid, cough aid
DOSAGE FORMS:
Tablets and Capsules:
25 mg, 50 mg; Chewable

tablets: 12.5 mg; Liquid, Solution, Elixir, and Syrup: 12.5 mg/5 mL; Cream: 1%, 2%

DIPIVEFRIN
dye PI ve frin
TRADE NAME(S):
Propine, AKPro
THERAPEUTIC CLASS:
Ocular agent
GENERAL USES:
Glaucoma
DOSAGE FORMS:
Ophthalmic solution: 0.1%

DIPYRIDAMOLE
dye peer ID a mole
TRADE NAME(S):
Persantine
THERAPEUTIC CLASS:
Antiplatelet agent
GENERAL USES:
Preventive therapy for blood clots
DOSAGE FORMS:
Tablets: 25 mg, 50 mg, 75 mg

DIRITHROMYCIN
dye RITH roe mye sin
TRADE NAME(S):
Dynabac
THERAPEUTIC CLASS:
Anti-infective
GENERAL USES:
Bacterial infections

DOSAGE FORMS:
Tablets: 250 mg

DISOPYRAMIDE
dye soe PEER a mide
TRADE NAME(S):
Norpace, Norpace CR
THERAPEUTIC CLASS:
Antiarrhythmic
GENERAL USES:
Ventricular arrhythmias
DOSAGE FORMS:
Capsules and Extended-release capsules: 100 mg, 150 mg

DISULFIRAM
dye SUL fi ram
TRADE NAME(S):
Antabuse
THERAPEUTIC CLASS:
Antialcoholic
GENERAL USES:
Alcohol abstinence
DOSAGE FORMS:
Tablets: 250 mg, 500 mg

DOBUTAMINE
doe BYOO ta meen
TRADE NAME(S):
Dobutrex
THERAPEUTIC CLASS:
Cardiac agent
GENERAL USES:
Increases cardiac contractility

DOSAGE FORMS:
Injection: 250 mg

DOCOSANOL
doe KOE san ole
TRADE NAME(S):
Abreva
THERAPEUTIC CLASS:
Antiviral
GENERAL USES:
Treatment of fever blisters, cold sores
DOSAGE FORMS:
Cream: 10%

DOFETILIDE
doe FET il ide
TRADE NAME(S):
Tikosyn
THERAPEUTIC CLASS:
Antiarrhythmic
GENERAL USES:
Atrial fibrillation/ flutter
DOSAGE FORMS:
Capsules: 125 mcg, 250 mcg, 500 mcg

DOLASETRON
dol A se tron
TRADE NAME(S):
Anzemet
THERAPEUTIC CLASS:
Antiemetic
GENERAL USES:
Surgical or chemotherapy nausea/vomiting

DOSAGE FORMS:
Tablets: 50 mg, 100 mg; Injection: 12.5 mg, 100 mg

DONEPEZIL
doh NEP e zil
TRADE NAME(S):
Aricept, Aricept ODT
THERAPEUTIC CLASS:
Alzheimer's agent
GENERAL USES:
Alzheimer's disease
DOSAGE FORMS:
Orally disintegrating tablets and Tablets: 5 mg, 10 mg

DOPAMINE
DOE pa meen
TRADE NAME(S):
Intropin
THERAPEUTIC CLASS:
Cardiac agent
GENERAL USES:
Increases cardiac output
DOSAGE FORMS:
Injection: 200 mg, 400 mg, 800 mg, 1.6 g

DORIPENEM
dore i PEN em
TRADE NAME(S):
Doribax
THERAPEUTIC CLASS:
Anti-infective
GENERAL USES:
Bacterial infection

DOSAGE FORMS:
  Injection: 500 mg

DORZOLAMIDE
dor ZOLE a mide
TRADE NAME(S):
  Trusopt
THERAPEUTIC CLASS:
  Ocular agent
GENERAL USES:
  Glaucoma/ocular
  hypertension
DOSAGE FORMS:
  Ophthalmic solution: 2%

**DORZOLAMIDE/
TIMOLOL**
dor ZOLE a mide/TYE moe
lole
TRADE NAME(S):
  Cosopt
THERAPEUTIC CLASS:
  Ocular agent
GENERAL USES:
  Glaucoma/ocular
  hypertension
DOSAGE FORMS:
  Ophthalmic solution:
  2%/0.5%

DOXAZOSIN
doks AY zoe sin
TRADE NAME(S):
  Cardura
THERAPEUTIC CLASS:
  Antihypertensive, BPH
  agent

GENERAL USES:
  Hypertension, BPH
DOSAGE FORMS:
  Tablets: 1 mg, 2 mg,
  4 mg, 8 mg

DOXEPIN (ORAL)
DOKS e pin
TRADE NAME(S):
  Sinequan
THERAPEUTIC CLASS:
  Antidepressant
GENERAL USES:
  Depression
DOSAGE FORMS:
  Capsules: 10 mg, 25 mg,
  50 mg, 75 mg, 100 mg,
  150 mg; Solution:
  10 mg/mL

DOXEPIN (TOPICAL)
DOKS e pin
TRADE NAME(S):
  Zonalon
THERAPEUTIC CLASS:
  Antipruritic (topical)
GENERAL USES:
  Pruritus
DOSAGE FORMS:
  Cream: 5%

DOXYCYCLINE
doks i SYE kleen
TRADE NAME(S):
  Vibramycin,
  Vibra-Tabs,
  Doxy, Doxychel

THERAPEUTIC CLASS:
Anti-infective

GENERAL USES:
Bacterial infections

DOSAGE FORMS:
Capsules: 20 mg, 50 mg,
100 mg; Tablets: 50 mg,
100 mg; Suspension:
25 mg/5 mL; Syrup:
50 mg/5 mL

DOXYCYCLINE
doks i SYE kleen
TRADE NAME(S):
Oracea
THERAPEUTIC CLASS:
Anti-infective
GENERAL USES:
Rosacea lesions
DOSAGE FORMS:
Capsules: 40 mg

DOXYCYCLINE
doks i SYE kleen
TRADE NAME(S):
Atridox
THERAPEUTIC CLASS:
Anti-infective
GENERAL USES:
Periodontitis
DOSAGE FORMS:
Oral gel: 10%

DRONABINOL
droe NAB i nol
TRADE NAME(S):
Marinol

THERAPEUTIC CLASS:
Antiemetic
GENERAL USES:
Chemotherapy nausea/
vomiting, appetite
stimulant
DOSAGE FORMS:
Capsules: 2.5 mg, 5 mg,
10 mg

DROTRECOGIN ALFA
dro TRE coe jin AL fa
TRADE NAME(S):
Xigris
THERAPEUTIC CLASS:
Biological
GENERAL USES:
Sepsis
DOSAGE FORMS:
Injection: 5 mg, 20 mg

DULOXETINE
doo LOKS e teen
TRADE NAME(S):
Cymbalta
THERAPEUTIC CLASS:
Antidepressant
GENERAL USES:
Depression, anxiety,
fibromyalgia
DOSAGE FORMS:
Delayed-release
capsules: 20 mg, 30 mg,
60 mg

DUTASTERIDE
doo TAS teer ide

TRADE NAME(S):
 Avodart
THERAPEUTIC CLASS:
 Antiandrogen
GENERAL USES:
 BPH
DOSAGE FORMS:
 Capsules: 0.5 mg

ECONAZOLE
e KONE a zole
TRADE NAME(S):
 Spectazole
THERAPEUTIC CLASS:
 Antifungal (topical)
GENERAL USES:
 Athlete's foot, jock itch,
 ringworm
DOSAGE FORMS:
 Cream: 1%

ECULIZUMAB
e kue LIZ oo mab
TRADE NAME(S):
 Soliris
THERAPEUTIC CLASS:
 Complement inhibitor
GENERAL USES:
 Nocturnal
 hemoglobinuria
DOSAGE FORMS:
 Injection: 300 mg

EFALIZUMAB
e fa li ZOO mab
TRADE NAME(S):
 Raptiva

THERAPEUTIC CLASS:
 Immunosuppressant
GENERAL USES:
 Psoriasis
DOSAGE FORMS:
 Injection: 125 mg

EFAVIRENZ
e FAV e renz
TRADE NAME(S):
 Sustiva
THERAPEUTIC CLASS:
 Antiviral
GENERAL USES:
 HIV infection
DOSAGE FORMS:
 Capsules: 50 mg, 100 mg,
 200 mg, 600 mg

EFAVIRENZ/ EMTRICITABINE/ TENOFOVIR DISOPROXIL FUMARATE
e FAV e renz/em trye SYE ta
been/te NOE fo veer
TRADE NAME(S):
 Atripla
THERAPEUTIC CLASS:
 Antiviral
GENERAL USES:
 HIV infection
DOSAGE FORMS:
 Tablets: 600 mg/200 mg/
 300 mg

ELETRIPTAN
el e TRIP tan

TRADE NAME(S):
  Relpax
THERAPEUTIC CLASS:
  Antimigraine
GENERAL USES:
  Migraines
DOSAGE FORMS:
  Tablets: 20 mg,
  40 mg

EMEDASTINE
em e DAS teen
TRADE NAME(S):
  Emadine
THERAPEUTIC CLASS:
  Ocular agent
GENERAL USES:
  Allergic conjunctivitis
DOSAGE FORMS:
  Ophthalmic solution:
  0.05%

EMTRICITABINE
em trye SYE ta been
TRADE NAME(S):
  Emtriva
THERAPEUTIC CLASS:
  Antiviral
GENERAL USES:
  HIV infection
DOSAGE FORMS:
  Capsules: 200 mg;
  Solution: 10 mg/mL

ENALAPRIL
e NAL a pril
TRADE NAME(S):
  Vasotec, Vasotec IV

THERAPEUTIC CLASS:
  Antihypertensive, cardiac
  agent
GENERAL USES:
  Hypertension, heart
  failure, left ventricular
  dysfunction
DOSAGE FORMS:
  Tablets: 2.5 mg, 5 mg,
  10 mg, 20 mg; Injection:
  1.25 mg, 2.5 mg
  (enalaprilat)

ENALAPRIL/HCTZ
e NAL a pril/hye droe klor oh
THYE a zide
TRADE NAME(S):
  Vaseretic
THERAPEUTIC CLASS:
  Antihypertensive/
  diuretic
GENERAL USES:
  Hypertension
DOSAGE FORMS:
  Tablets: 5 mg/12.5 mg,
  10 mg/25 mg

ENFUVIRTIDE
en FYOO vir tide
TRADE NAME(S):
  Fuzeon
THERAPEUTIC CLASS:
  Antiviral
GENERAL USES:
  HIV infection
DOSAGE FORMS:
  Injection: 90 mg

ENOXACIN
en OKS a sin
TRADE NAME(S):
Penetrex
THERAPEUTIC CLASS:
Anti-infective
GENERAL USES:
Bacterial infections
DOSAGE FORMS:
Tablets: 200 mg, 400 mg

ENOXAPARIN SODIUM
ee noks a PA rin
TRADE NAME(S):
Lovenox
THERAPEUTIC CLASS:
Anticoagulant (LMWH)
GENERAL USES:
Prevention of blood clots
DOSAGE FORMS:
Injection: 30 mg, 40 mg,
60 mg, 80 mg, 90 mg,
100 mg, 120 mg, 150 mg

ENTACAPONE
en TA ka pone
TRADE NAME(S):
Comtan
THERAPEUTIC CLASS:
Antiparkinson agent
GENERAL USES:
Parkinson's disease
DOSAGE FORMS:
Tablets: 200 mg

ENTECAVIR
en TE ka veer
TRADE NAME(S):
Baraclude
THERAPEUTIC CLASS:
Antiviral
GENERAL USES:
Chronic hepatitis B
DOSAGE FORMS:
Solution: 0.05 mg/mL;
Tablets: 0.5 mg, 1 mg

EPINASTINE (OCULAR)
ep i NAS teen
TRADE NAME(S):
Elestat
THERAPEUTIC CLASS:
Ocular (antihistamine)
GENERAL USES:
Allergic conjunctivitis
DOSAGE FORMS:
Ophthalmic solution:
0.05%

EPINEPHRINE
ep i NEF rin
TRADE NAME(S):
Epifrin, Glaucon
THERAPEUTIC CLASS:
Ocular agent
GENERAL USES:
Glaucoma
DOSAGE FORMS:
Ophthalmic solution:
0.1%, 0.5%, 1%, 2%

EPLERENONE
e PLER en one
TRADE NAME(S):
Inspra

THERAPEUTIC CLASS:
Antihypertensive
GENERAL USES:
Hypertension
DOSAGE FORMS:
Tablets: 25 mg, 50 mg,
100 mg

EPOETIN ALFA
e POE e tin
TRADE NAME(S):
Epogen, Procrit
THERAPEUTIC CLASS:
Hematological agent
GENERAL USES:
Anemia with chronic renal
failure, cancer, or HIV
infection
DOSAGE FORMS:
Injection: 2000 units,
3000 units, 4000 units,
10,000 units, 20,000 units

ERGOTAMINE TARTRATE
er GOT a meen
TRADE NAME(S):
Ergomar
THERAPEUTIC CLASS:
Antimigraine agent
GENERAL USES:
Migraines
DOSAGE FORMS:
Sublingual tablets:
2 mg

ERLOTINIB
er LOE tye nib

TRADE NAME(S):
Tarceva
THERAPEUTIC CLASS:
EGFR inhibitor
GENERAL USES:
Non-small-cell lung
cancer, pancreatic cancer
DOSAGE FORMS:
Tablets: 25 mg, 100 mg,
150 mg

ERTAPENEM
er ta PEN em
TRADE NAME(S):
Invanz
THERAPEUTIC CLASS:
Anti-infective
GENERAL USES:
Bacterial infections
DOSAGE FORMS:
Injection: 1 g

ERYTHROMYCIN (BASE)
er ith roe MYE sin
TRADE NAME(S):
E-Mycin, E-Base, PCE,
Ery-Tab, Eryc
THERAPEUTIC CLASS:
Anti-infective
GENERAL USES:
Bacterial infections
DOSAGE FORMS:
Tablets: 250 mg, 333 mg,
500 mg; Delayed-release
capsules: 250 mg

ERYTHROMYCIN (OCULAR)

er ith roe MYE sin

TRADE NAME(S):
Ilotycin

THERAPEUTIC CLASS:
Ocular agent (anti-infective)

GENERAL USES:
Ocular infections

DOSAGE FORMS:
Ophthalmic ointment: 5%

ERYTHROMYCIN (TOPICAL)

er ith roe MYE sin

TRADE NAME(S):
Akne-mycin, Emgel, Erygel

THERAPEUTIC CLASS:
Anti-infective (topical)

GENERAL USES:
Acne

DOSAGE FORMS:
Ointment and Gel: 2%; Solution: 1.5%, 2%

ERYTHROMYCIN ESTOLATE

er ith roe MYE sin

TRADE NAME(S):
Ilosone

THERAPEUTIC CLASS:
Anti-infective

GENERAL USES:
Bacterial infections

DOSAGE FORMS:
Tablets: 500 mg; Capsules: 250 mg; Suspension: 125 mg/ 5 mL, 250 mg/5 mL

ERYTHROMYCIN ETHYLSUCCINATE

er ith roe MYE sin

TRADE NAME(S):
EryPed, EES

THERAPEUTIC CLASS:
Anti-infective

GENERAL USES:
Bacterial infections

DOSAGE FORMS:
Tablets: 400 mg; Chewable tablets: 200 mg; Suspension: 200 mg/5 mL, 400 mg/ 5 mL, 100 mg/2.5 mL

ERYTHROMYCIN LACTOBIONATE

er ith roe MYE sin

TRADE NAME(S):
Erythrocin

THERAPEUTIC CLASS:
Anti-infective

GENERAL USES:
Bacterial infections

DOSAGE FORMS:
Injection: 500 mg, 1 g

ERYTHROMYCIN STEARATE

er ith roe MYE sin

TRADE NAME(S):
Erythrocin

THERAPEUTIC CLASS:
Anti-infective

GENERAL USES:
Bacterial infections

DOSAGE FORMS:
Tablets: 250 mg, 500 mg

ERYTHROMYCIN/ BENZOYL PEROXIDE
er ith roe MYE sin/BEN zoyl per OKS ide

TRADE NAME(S):
Benzamycin

THERAPEUTIC CLASS:
Anti-infective (topical)

GENERAL USES:
Acne

DOSAGE FORMS:
Gel: 30 mg/50 mg per g

ESCITALOPRAM
es sye TAL oh pram

TRADE NAME(S):
Lexapro

THERAPEUTIC CLASS:
Antidepressant

GENERAL USES:
Depression, anxiety

DOSAGE FORMS:
Tablets: 5 mg, 10 mg, 20 mg; Solution: 1 mg/ mL

ESOMEPRAZOLE
es oh ME pray zol

TRADE NAME(S):
Nexium

THERAPEUTIC CLASS:
Gastric acid secretion inhibitor

GENERAL USES:
GERD, erosive esophagitis, Zollinger-Ellison syndrome

DOSAGE FORMS:
Injection and capsules: 20 mg, 40 mg

ESTAZOLAM
es TA zoe lam

TRADE NAME(S):
ProSom

THERAPEUTIC CLASS:
Sedative/hypnotic

GENERAL USES:
Insomnia

DOSAGE FORMS:
Tablets: 1 mg, 2 mg

ESTRADIOL (GEL)
es tra DYE ole

TRADE NAME(S):
EstroGel, Divigel

THERAPEUTIC CLASS:
Hormone (estrogen)

GENERAL USES:
Vasomotor symptoms of menopause

DOSAGE FORMS:
Gel/Pump: 0.06%; Gel: 0.1%

ESTRADIOL (SPRAY)
es tra DYE ole

Trade Name(s):
Evamist

Therapeutic Class:
Hormone (estrogen)

General Uses:
Estrogen replacement

Dosage Forms:
Spray: 1.53 mg/spray

ESTRADIOL (TRANSDERMAL)
es tra DYE ole

Trade Name(s):
FemPatch, Vivelle, Alora, Estraderm, Climara, Menostar, Vivelle-Dot

Therapeutic Class:
Hormone (estrogen)

General Uses:
Estrogen replacement

Dosage Forms:
Transdermal patch (release rate/24 hr): 0.014 mg, 0.025 mg, 0.0375 mg, 0.05 mg, 0.075 mg, 0.1 mg

ESTRADIOL (VAGINAL RING)
es tra DYE ole

Trade Name(s):
Femring

Therapeutic Class:
Hormone (estrogen)

General Uses:
Vasomotor symptoms of menopause

Dosage Forms:
Vaginal ring: 0.05 mg/day, 0.1 mg/day

ESTRADIOL, 17-BETA (TOPICAL EMULSION)
es tra DYE ole

Trade Name(s):
Estrasorb

Therapeutic Class:
Hormone (estrogen)

General Uses:
Estrogen replacement

Dosage Forms:
Topical emulsion pouch: 1.74 g (4.35 mg estradiol)

ESTRADIOL/ DROSPIRENONE
es tra DYE ole/droh SPYE re none

Trade Name(s):
Angeliq

Therapeutic Class:
Hormone

General Uses:
Menopausal symptoms

Dosage Forms:
Tablets: 1 mg/0.5 mg

ESTRADIOL/ LEVONORGESTREL (TRANSDERMAL)
es tra DYE ole/LEE voe nor

jes trel

TRADE NAME(S):
Climara Pro

THERAPEUTIC CLASS:
Hormone (estrogen/
progestin)

GENERAL USES:
Vasomotor symptoms of
menopause

DOSAGE FORMS:
Patch: 45 mcg/15 mcg

ESTRADIOL/ NORETHINDRONE
es tra DYE ole/nor
eth IN drone

TRADE NAME(S):
Activella

THERAPEUTIC CLASS:
Hormone
(estrogen/
progestin)

GENERAL USES:
Estrogen
replacement

DOSAGE FORMS:
Tablets: 1 mg/0.5 mg

ESTROGENS, CONJUGATED
ES troe jenz

TRADE NAME(S):
Premarin, Premarin IV

THERAPEUTIC CLASS:
Hormone (estrogen)

GENERAL USES:
Estrogen replacement

DOSAGE FORMS:
Tablets: 0.3 mg,
0.625 mg, 0.9 mg,
1.25 mg, 2.5 mg;
Injection: 25 mg

ESTROGENS, ESTERIFIED
ES troe jenz, es TER i fied

TRADE NAME(S):
Estratab, Menest

THERAPEUTIC CLASS:
Hormone (estrogen)

GENERAL USES:
Estrogen replacement

DOSAGE FORMS:
Tablets: 0.3 mg,
0.625 mg, 1.25 mg,
2.5 mg

ESTROGENS A, CONJUGATED (SYNTHETIC)
ES troe jenz

TRADE NAME(S):
Cenestin

THERAPEUTIC CLASS:
Hormone

GENERAL USES:
Vasomotor symptoms
of menopause, vaginal
atrophy

DOSAGE FORMS:
Tablets: 0.3 mg,
0.625 mg, 0.9 mg,
1.25 mg

ESTROGENS B, CONJUGATED (SYNTHETIC)
ES troe jenz

TRADE NAME(S):
Enjuvia

THERAPEUTIC CLASS:
Hormone

GENERAL USES:
Vasomotor symptoms of menopause

DOSAGE FORMS:
Tablets: 0.625 mg, 1.25 mg

ESTROGENS, CONJUGATED/ MEDROXY-PROGESTERONE
ES troe jenz/me DROKS ee proe JES te rone

TRADE NAME(S):
Prempro, Premphase

THERAPEUTIC CLASS:
Hormone (estrogen/ progestin)

GENERAL USES:
Estrogen replacement

DOSAGE FORMS:
Tablets: 0.625 mg/5 mg, 0.625 mg/2.5 mg, 0.3 mg/1.5 mg, 0.45 mg/ 1.5 mg

ESTROPIPATE
ES troe pih pate

TRADE NAME(S):
Ogen, Ortho-Est

THERAPEUTIC CLASS:
Hormone (estrogen)

GENERAL USES:
Estrogen replacement

DOSAGE FORMS:
Tablets: 0.625 mg, 1.25 mg, 2.5 mg, 5 mg; Vaginal cream: 0.15%

ESZOPICLONE
es zoe PIK lone

TRADE NAME(S):
Lunesta

THERAPEUTIC CLASS:
Hypnotic

GENERAL USES:
Insomnia

DOSAGE FORMS:
Tablets: 1 mg, 2 mg, 3 mg

ETANERCEPT
et a NER sept

TRADE NAME(S):
Enbrel

THERAPEUTIC CLASS:
Immunomodulator

GENERAL USES:
Rheumatoid and psoriatic arthritis, plaque psoriasis, ankylosing spondylitis

DOSAGE FORMS:
Injection: 25 mg, 50 mg

ETHACRYNIC ACID
eth a KRIN ik AS id

TRADE NAME(S):
Edecrin

THERAPEUTIC CLASS:
Diuretic

GENERAL USES:
CHF-related edema,
hypertension

DOSAGE FORMS:
Tablets: 25 mg, 50 mg

ETHAMBUTOL
e THAM byoo tole

TRADE NAME(S):
Myambutol

THERAPEUTIC CLASS:
Antituberculosis agent

GENERAL USES:
Tuberculosis

DOSAGE FORMS:
Tablets: 100 mg, 400 mg

ETHINYL ESTRADIOL
ETH in il es tra DYE ole

TRADE NAME(S):
Estinyl

THERAPEUTIC CLASS:
Hormone (estrogen)

GENERAL USES:
Estrogen
replacement

DOSAGE FORMS:
Tablets: 0.02 mg,
0.05 mg, 0.25 mg,
0.5 mg

ETHINYL ESTRADIOL/ DESOGESTREL
ETH in il es tra DYE ole/des
oh JES trel

TRADE NAME(S):
Desogen, Ortho-Cept,
Apri

THERAPEUTIC CLASS:
Contraceptive
(monophasic)

GENERAL USES:
Contraception

DOSAGE FORMS:
Tablets: 30 mcg/0.15 mg

ETHINYL ESTRADIOL/ DESOGESTREL
ETH in il es tra DYE ole/des
oh JES trel

TRADE NAME(S):
Mircette, Kariva

THERAPEUTIC CLASS:
Contraceptive (biphasic)

GENERAL USES:
Contraception

DOSAGE FORMS:
Tablets: Phase 1: 20 mcg/
0.15 mg; Phase 2: 10 mcg
(EE)

ETHINYL ESTRADIOL/ DROSPIRENONE
ETH in il es tra DYE ole/droh
SPYE re none

TRADE NAME(S):
Yasmin

THERAPEUTIC CLASS:
Contraceptive
(monophasic)
GENERAL USES:
Contraception
DOSAGE FORMS:
Tablets: 0.03 mg/3 mg

ETHINYL ESTRADIOL/ DROSPIRENONE
ETH in il es tra DYE ole/droh SPYE re none
TRADE NAME(S):
Yaz
THERAPEUTIC CLASS:
Contraceptive
GENERAL USES:
Contraception, PMDD
DOSAGE FORMS:
Tablets: 20 mcg/3 mg

ETHINYL ESTRADIOL/ ETHYNODIOL
ETH in il es tra DYE ole/e thye noe DYE ole
TRADE NAME(S):
Demulen 1/50, Zovia 1/50E
THERAPEUTIC CLASS:
Contraceptive
(monophasic)
GENERAL USES:
Contraception
DOSAGE FORMS:
Tablets: 50 mcg/1 mg

ETHINYL ESTRADIOL/ ETHYNODIOL
ETH in il es tra DYE ole/e thye noe DYE ole
TRADE NAME(S):
Demulen 1/35, Zovia 1/35E
THERAPEUTIC CLASS:
Contraceptive
(monophasic)
GENERAL USES:
Contraception
DOSAGE FORMS:
Tablets: 35 mcg/1 mg

ETHINYL ESTRADIOL/ ETONOGESTREL
ETH in il es tra DYE ole/et oh noe JES trel
TRADE NAME(S):
NuvaRing
THERAPEUTIC CLASS:
Contraceptive
GENERAL USES:
Contraception
DOSAGE FORMS:
Vaginal ring (release rate/ 24 hr): 15 mcg/120 mcg

ETHINYL ESTRADIOL/ LEVONORGESTREL
ETH in il es tra DYE ole/LEE voe nor jes trel
TRADE NAME(S):
Preven
THERAPEUTIC CLASS:
Contraceptive
(emergency)

GENERAL USES:
Emergency contraception
DOSAGE FORMS:
Tablets: 50 mcg/0.25 mg

**ETHINYL ESTRADIOL/
LEVONORGESTREL**
ETH in il es tra DYE ole/LEE
voe nor jes trel
TRADE NAME(S):
Seasonique
THERAPEUTIC CLASS:
Contraceptive
GENERAL USES:
Contraception
DOSAGE FORMS:
Tablets: 30 mcg/15 mcg,
10 mcg/15 mcg

**ETHINYL ESTRADIOL/
LEVONORGESTREL**
ETH in il es tra DYE ole/LEE
voe nor jes trel
TRADE NAME(S):
Levlen, Levora 0.15/30,
Nordette, Portia
THERAPEUTIC CLASS:
Contraceptive
(monophasic)
GENERAL USES:
Contraception
DOSAGE FORMS:
Tablets: 30 mcg/0.15 mg

**ETHINYL ESTRADIOL/
LEVONORGESTREL**
ETH in il es tra DYE ole/LEE

voe nor jes trel
TRADE NAME(S):
Seasonale
THERAPEUTIC CLASS:
Hormone (estrogen/
progestin)
GENERAL USES:
Contraception
(91-day regimen)
DOSAGE FORMS:
Tablets: 30 mcg/150 mcg

**ETHINYL ESTRADIOL/
LEVONORGESTREL**
ETH in il es tra DYE ole/LEE
voe nor jes trel
TRADE NAME(S):
Levlite, Alesse, Lessina,
Aviane
THERAPEUTIC CLASS:
Contraceptive
(monophasic)
GENERAL USES:
Contraception
DOSAGE FORMS:
Tablets: 20 mcg/0.1 mg

**ETHINYL ESTRADIOL/
LEVONORGESTREL**
ETH in il es tra DYE ole/LEE
voe nor jes trel
TRADE NAME(S):
Lybrel
THERAPEUTIC CLASS:
Contraceptive
GENERAL USES:
Contraception

DOSAGE FORMS:
Tablets: 20 mcg/90 mcg

ETHINYL ESTRADIOL/ LEVONORGESTREL

ETH in il es tra DYE ole/LEE voe nor jes trel

TRADE NAME(S):
Enpresse, Tri-Levlen, Triphasil, Trivora-28

THERAPEUTIC CLASS:
Contraceptive (triphasic)

GENERAL USES:
Contraception

DOSAGE FORMS:
Tablets: Phase 1: 30 mcg/0.05 mg; Phase 2: 40 mcg/ 0.075 mg; Phase 3: 30 mcg/ 0.125 mg

ETHINYL ESTRADIOL/ NORELGESTROMIN

ETH in il es tra DYE ole/nor el JES troe min

TRADE NAME(S):
Ortho Evra

THERAPEUTIC CLASS:
Contraceptive

GENERAL USES:
Contraception

DOSAGE FORMS:
Transdermal patch (release rate/24 hr): 20 mcg/150 mcg

ETHINYL ESTRADIOL/ NORETHINDRONE

ETH in il es tra DYE ole/nor eth IN drone

TRADE NAME(S):
Ovcon 50

THERAPEUTIC CLASS:
Contraceptive (monophasic)

GENERAL USES:
Contraception

DOSAGE FORMS:
Tablets: 50 mcg/1 mg

ETHINYL ESTRADIOL/ NORETHINDRONE

ETH in il es tra DYE ole/nor eth IN drone

TRADE NAME(S):
Genora 1/35, Nelova 1/35E, Norethin 1/35E, Norinyl 1+35, Nortrel 1/35, Necon 1/35, Ortho-Novum 1/35

THERAPEUTIC CLASS:
Contraceptive (monophasic)

GENERAL USES:
Contraception

DOSAGE FORMS:
Tablets: 35 mcg/1 mg

ETHINYL ESTRADIOL/ NORETHINDRONE

ETH in il es tra DYE ole/nor eth IN drone

TRADE NAME(S):
Brevicon, Modicon,

Genora 0.5/35, Nelova
0.5/35E, Necon 0.5/35,
Nortrel 0.5/35
THERAPEUTIC CLASS:
Contraceptive
(monophasic)
GENERAL USES:
Contraception
DOSAGE FORMS:
Tablets: 35 mcg/0.5 mg

**ETHINYL ESTRADIOL/
NORETHINDRONE**
ETH in il es tra DYE ole/nor
eth IN drone
TRADE NAME(S):
Ovcon 35
THERAPEUTIC CLASS:
Contraceptive
(monophasic)
GENERAL USES:
Contraception
DOSAGE FORMS:
Chewable tablets and
Tablets: 35 mcg/
0.4 mg

**ETHINYL ESTRADIOL/
NORETHINDRONE**
ETH in il es tra DYE ole/nor
eth IN drone
TRADE NAME(S):
Loestrin 1.5/30,
Microgestin 1.5/30
THERAPEUTIC CLASS:
Contraceptive
(monophasic)

GENERAL USES:
Contraception
DOSAGE FORMS:
Tablets: 30 mcg/
1.5 mg

**ETHINYL ESTRADIOL/
NORETHINDRONE**
ETH in il es tra DYE ole/nor
eth IN drone
TRADE NAME(S):
Loestrin 1/20, Loestrin Fe
1/20, Microgestin Fe 1/20
THERAPEUTIC CLASS:
Contraceptive
(monophasic)
GENERAL USES:
Contraception
DOSAGE FORMS:
Tablets: 20 mcg/1 mg

**ETHINYL ESTRADIOL/
NORETHINDRONE**
ETH in il es tra DYE ole/nor
eth IN drone
TRADE NAME(S):
Jenest-28, Nelova 10/11,
Ortho-Novum 10/11,
Necon 10/11
THERAPEUTIC CLASS:
Contraceptive (biphasic)
GENERAL USES:
Contraception
DOSAGE FORMS:
Tablets: Phase 1:
35 mcg/0.5 mg; Phase 2:
35 mcg/1 mg

ETHINYL ESTRADIOL/ NORETHINDRONE

ETH in il es tra DYE ole/nor eth IN drone

TRADE NAME(S):
Tri-Norinyl

THERAPEUTIC CLASS:
Contraceptive (triphasic)

GENERAL USES:
Contraception

DOSAGE FORMS:
Tablets: Phase 1:
35 mcg/0.5 mg; Phase 2:
35 mcg/1 mg; Phase 3:
35 mcg/0.5 mg

ETHINYL ESTRADIOL/ NORETHINDRONE

ETH in il es tra DYE ole/nor eth IN drone

TRADE NAME(S):
Ortho-Novum 7/7/7,
Necon 7/7/7

THERAPEUTIC CLASS:
Contraceptive (triphasic)

GENERAL USES:
Contraception

DOSAGE FORMS:
Tablets: Phase 1:
35 mcg/0.5 mg; Phase 2:
35 mcg/0.75 mg; Phase
3: 35 mcg/1 mg

ETHINYL ESTRADIOL/ NORETHINDRONE

ETH in il es tra DYE ole/nor eth IN drone

TRADE NAME(S):
Estrostep, Estrostep Fe

THERAPEUTIC CLASS:
Contraceptive (triphasic)

GENERAL USES:
Contraception

DOSAGE FORMS:
Tablets: Phase 1:
20 mcg/1 mg; Phase 2:
30 mcg/1 mg; Phase 3:
35 mcg/1 mg

ETHINYL ESTRADIOL/ NORGESTIMATE

ETH in il es tra DYE ole/nor JES ti mate

TRADE NAME(S):
Ortho-Cyclen, Sprintec

THERAPEUTIC CLASS:
Contraceptive
(monophasic)

GENERAL USES:
Contraception

DOSAGE FORMS:
Tablets: 35 mcg/0.25 mg

ETHINYL ESTRADIOL/ NORGESTIMATE

ETH in il es tra DYE ole/nor JES ti mate

TRADE NAME(S):
Ortho-Tri-Cyclen

THERAPEUTIC CLASS:
Contraceptive
(triphasic)

GENERAL USES:
Contraception

DOSAGE FORMS:
Tablets: Phase 1:
35 mcg/0.18 mg; Phase 2:
35 mcg/0.215 mg; Phase
3: 35 mcg/0.25 mg

ETHINYL ESTRADIOL/ NORGESTREL
ETH in il es tra DYE ole/nor
JES trel
TRADE NAME(S):
Ovral, Ogestrel
THERAPEUTIC CLASS:
Contraceptive
(monophasic)
GENERAL USES:
Contraception
DOSAGE FORMS:
Tablets: 50 mcg/0.5 mg

ETHINYL ESTRADIOL/ NORGESTREL
ETH in il es tra DYE ole/nor
JES trel
TRADE NAME(S):
Cryselle, Lo/Ovral, Low-
Ogestrel
THERAPEUTIC CLASS:
Contraceptive
(monophasic)
GENERAL USES:
Contraception
DOSAGE FORMS:
Tablets: 30 mcg/0.3 mg

ETHIONAMIDE
e thye on AM ide

TRADE NAME(S):
Trecator-SC
THERAPEUTIC CLASS:
Antituberculosis agent
GENERAL USES:
Tuberculosis
DOSAGE FORMS:
Tablets: 250 mg

ETHOSUXIMIDE
eth oh SUKS i mide
TRADE NAME(S):
Zarontin
THERAPEUTIC CLASS:
Anticonvulsant
GENERAL USES:
Seizures
DOSAGE FORMS:
Capsules: 250 mg; Syrup:
250 mg/5 mL

ETIDRONATE
e ti DROE nate
TRADE NAME(S):
Didronel
THERAPEUTIC CLASS:
Bisphosphonate
GENERAL USES:
Paget's disease,
hypercalcemia (cancer
related)
DOSAGE FORMS:
Tablets: 200 mg,
400 mg

ETODOLAC
ee toe DOE lak

Trade Name(s):
Lodine, Lodine XL

Therapeutic Class:
Anti-inflammatory/
analgesic

General Uses:
Osteoarthritis, rheumatoid
arthritis, ankylosing
spondylitis, pain

Dosage Forms:
Tablets: 400 mg, 500 mg;
Extended-release tablets:
400 mg, 500 mg, 600 mg;
Capsules: 200 mg,
300 mg

ETONOGESTREL
et oh noe JES trel

Trade Name(s):
Implanon

Therapeutic Class:
Contraceptive

General Uses:
Contraception

Dosage Forms:
Implant: 68 mg

ETRAVIRINE
e tra VIR een

Trade Name(s):
Intelence

Therapeutic Class:
Antiviral

General Uses:
HIV infection

Dosage Forms:
Tablets: 100 mg

ETRETINATE
ee TRET ih nate

Trade Name(s):
Tegison

Therapeutic Class:
Retinoid

General Uses:
Psoriasis

Dosage Forms:
Capsules: 10 mg, 25 mg

EXEMESTANE
ex e MES tane

Trade Name(s):
Aromasin

Therapeutic Class:
Antineoplastic

General Uses:
Breast cancer

Dosage Forms:
Tablets: 25 mg

EXENATIDE
eks EN a tide

Trade Name(s):
Byetta

Therapeutic Class:
Antidiabetic

General Uses:
Diabetes

Dosage Forms:
Injection: 250 mcg/mL

EZETIMIBE
ez ET i mibe

Trade Name(s):
Zetia

THERAPEUTIC CLASS:
Antilipemic
GENERAL USES:
Hyperlipidemia
DOSAGE FORMS:
Tablets: 10 mg

**EZETIMIBE/
SIMVASTATIN**
ez ET i mibe/SIM va stat in
TRADE NAME(S):
Vytorin
THERAPEUTIC CLASS:
Antilipemic
GENERAL USES:
Hypercholesterolemia
DOSAGE FORMS:
Tablets: 10 mg/10 mg,
10 mg/20 mg, 10 mg/
40 mg, 10 mg/80 mg

FAMCICLOVIR
fam SYE kloe veer
TRADE NAME(S):
Famvir
THERAPEUTIC CLASS:
Antiviral
GENERAL USES:
Herpes, shingles
DOSAGE FORMS:
Tablets: 125 mg, 250 mg,
500 mg

FAMOTIDINE
fa MOE ti deen
TRADE NAME(S):
Pepcid, Pepcid AC,
Pepcid RPD
THERAPEUTIC CLASS:
Gastric acid secretion
inhibitor
GENERAL USES:
GERD, GI ulcers
DOSAGE FORMS:
Tablets: 10 mg, 20 mg,
40 mg; Chewable tablets:
10 mg; Suspension:
40 mg/5 mL; Injection:
20 mg, 40 mg

FELODIPINE
fe LOE di peen
TRADE NAME(S):
Plendil
THERAPEUTIC CLASS:
Antihypertensive
GENERAL USES:
Hypertension
DOSAGE FORMS:
Extended-release tablets:
2.5 mg, 5 mg, 10 mg

FENOFIBRATE
fen oh FYE brate
TRADE NAME(S):
TriCor, Antara, Triglide,
Lipofen
THERAPEUTIC CLASS:
Antilipemic
GENERAL USES:
Hyperlipidemia
DOSAGE FORMS:
Capsules: 43 mg, 50 mg,
67 mg, 87 mg, 130 mg,

134 mg, 150 mg, 200 mg;
Tablets: 48 mg, 50 mg,
145 mg

FENOPROFEN
fen oh PROE fen
TRADE NAME(S):
Nalfon
THERAPEUTIC CLASS:
Anti-inflammatory/
analgesic
GENERAL USES:
Osteoarthritis, rheumatoid
arthritis, pain
DOSAGE FORMS:
Capsules: 200 mg,
300 mg; Tablets: 600 mg

FENTANYL (BUCCAL)
FEN ta nil
TRADE NAME(S):
Fentora
THERAPEUTIC CLASS:
Analgesic (narcotic)
GENERAL USES:
Pain
DOSAGE FORMS:
Buccal tablets: 100 mcg,
200 mcg, 400 mcg,
600 mcg, 800 mcg

FENTANYL (INJECTION)
FEN ta nil
TRADE NAME(S):
Sublimaze
THERAPEUTIC CLASS:
Analgesic (narcotic)

GENERAL USES:
Premedicant for
anesthesia
DOSAGE FORMS:
Injection: 0.1 mg,
0.25 mg, 0.5 mg, 1 mg,
1.5 mg, 2.5 mg

FENTANYL (ORAL)
FEN ta nil
TRADE NAME(S):
Actiq, Oralet
THERAPEUTIC CLASS:
Analgesic (narcotic)
GENERAL USES:
Pain, pre-op medication
DOSAGE FORMS:
Lozenge: 200 mcg,
300 mcg, 400 mcg;
Lozenge/stick: 200 mcg,
400 mcg, 600 mcg,
800 mcg, 1200 mcg,
1600 mcg

**FENTANYL
(TRANSDERMAL)**
FEN ta nil
TRADE NAME(S):
Duragesic
THERAPEUTIC CLASS:
Analgesic (narcotic)
GENERAL USES:
Pain
DOSAGE FORMS:
Transdermal patch (mcg/
hr): 25, 50, 75, 100

FEXOFENADINE
feks oh FEN a deen
TRADE NAME(S):
Allegra
THERAPEUTIC CLASS:
Antihistamine
GENERAL USES:
Allergic rhinitis, chronic
hives
DOSAGE FORMS:
Tablets: 30 mg, 60 mg,
180 mg; Oral suspension:
6 mg/mL

**FEXOFENADINE/
PSEUDOEPHEDRINE**
feks oh FEN a deen/soo doe
e FED rin
TRADE NAME(S):
Allegra-D 12 Hour,
Allegra-D 24 Hour
THERAPEUTIC CLASS:
Antihistamine/
decongestant
GENERAL USES:
Allergic rhinitis
DOSAGE FORMS:
Extended-release tablets:
60 mg/120 mg,
180 mg/240 mg

FINASTERIDE
fi NAS teer ide
TRADE NAME(S):
Propecia, Proscar
THERAPEUTIC CLASS:
Antiandrogen

GENERAL USES:
Male-pattern baldness,
BPH
DOSAGE FORMS:
Tablets: 1 mg, 5 mg

FLECAINIDE
fle KAY nide
TRADE NAME(S):
Tambocor
THERAPEUTIC CLASS:
Antiarrhythmic
GENERAL USES:
Atrial fibrillation,
tachycardia, arrhythmias
DOSAGE FORMS:
Tablets: 50 mg, 100 mg,
150 mg

FLUCONAZOLE
floo KOE na zole
TRADE NAME(S):
Diflucan, Diflucan IV
THERAPEUTIC CLASS:
Antifungal
GENERAL USES:
Fungal infections
DOSAGE FORMS:
Tablets: 50 mg, 100 mg,
150 mg, 200 mg;
Suspension: 10 mg/mL,
40 mg/mL; Injection:
200 mg, 400 mg

FLUCYTOSINE
floo SYE toe seen
TRADE NAME(S):
Ancobon

THERAPEUTIC CLASS:
Antifungal
GENERAL USES:
Fungal infections
DOSAGE FORMS:
Capsules: 250 mg,
500 mg

FLUNISOLIDE (INHALED)
floo NISS oh lide
TRADE NAME(S):
AeroBid
THERAPEUTIC CLASS:
Corticosteroid (inhaler)
GENERAL USES:
Asthma (chronic)
DOSAGE FORMS:
Inhaler: 250 mcg/
inhalation

FLUNISOLIDE (NASAL)
floo NISS oh lide
TRADE NAME(S):
Nasalide, Nasarel
THERAPEUTIC CLASS:
Corticosteroid (nasal)
GENERAL USES:
Allergies
DOSAGE FORMS:
Nasal spray: 0.025%

FLUOCINOLONE
floo oh SIN oh lone
TRADE NAME(S):
Synalar, Fluonid, Flurosyn
THERAPEUTIC CLASS:
Corticosteroid (topical)

GENERAL USES:
Various skin
conditions
DOSAGE FORMS:
Ointment: 0.025%;
Cream: 0.01%, 0.025%,
0.2%; Solution: 0.01%

FLUOCINOLONE ACETONIDE (IMPLANT)
floo oh SIN oh lone ah SEE
toe nide
TRADE NAME(S):
Retisert
THERAPEUTIC CLASS:
Ocular agent
GENERAL USES:
Noninfectious
uveitis
DOSAGE FORMS:
Intravitreal implant:
0.59 mg

FLUOCINONIDE
floo oh SIN oh nide
TRADE NAME(S):
Lidex, Fluonex, Vanos
THERAPEUTIC CLASS:
Corticosteroid (topical)
GENERAL USES:
Various skin conditions
DOSAGE FORMS:
Cream, Ointment,
Solution, and Gel: 0.05%;
Cream: 0.1%

FLUOROMETHOLONE
flure oh METH oh lone

Trade Name(s):
Fluor-Op, FML, Flarex
Therapeutic Class:
Ocular agent (steroid)
General Uses:
Ocular inflammation
Dosage Forms:
Ophthalmic
suspension: 0.1%, 0.25%;
Ophthalmic ointment:
0.1%

FLUOROURACIL
(INJECTION)
flure oh YOOR a sil
Trade Name(s):
Adrucil, 5-FU
Therapeutic Class:
Antineoplastic
General Uses:
Cancers of the colon,
rectum, breast,
stomach, and
pancreas
Dosage Forms:
Injection: 500 mg, 1 g,
2.5 g, 5 g

FLUOROURACIL
(TOPICAL)
flure oh YOOR a sil
Trade Name(s):
Efudex, Fluoroplex
Therapeutic Class:
Antineoplastic
General Uses:
Skin disorders

Dosage Forms:
Cream: 1%, 5%; Solution:
1%, 2%, 5%

FLUOXETINE
floo OKS e teen
Trade Name(s):
Prozac, Prozac Weekly,
Sarafem
Therapeutic Class:
Antidepressant
General Uses:
Depression, bulimia, OCD,
PMDD
Dosage Forms:
Capsules: 10 mg, 20 mg,
40 mg; Solution: 20 mg/
5 mL; Delayed-release
capsules: 90 mg

FLUPHENAZINE
floo FEN a zeen
Trade Name(s):
Prolixin, Permitil
Therapeutic Class:
Antipsychotic
General Uses:
Psychotic disorders
Dosage Forms:
Tablets: 1 mg,
2.5 mg, 5 mg, 10 mg;
Elixir: 2.5 mg/5 mL;
Concentrated solution:
5 mg/mL

FLURAZEPAM
flure AZ e pam

TRADE NAME(S):
Dalmane

THERAPEUTIC CLASS:
Sedative/hypnotic

GENERAL USES:
Insomnia

DOSAGE FORMS:
Capsules: 15 mg, 30 mg

FLURBIPROFEN (OCULAR)
flur BI proe fen

TRADE NAME(S):
Ocufen

THERAPEUTIC CLASS:
Ocular agent

GENERAL USES:
Maintain pupil dilation during surgery

DOSAGE FORMS:
Ophthalmic solution: 0.03%

FLURBIPROFEN (ORAL)
flur BI proe fen

TRADE NAME(S):
Ansaid

THERAPEUTIC CLASS:
Anti-inflammatory/ analgesic

GENERAL USES:
Osteoarthritis, rheumatoid arthritis

DOSAGE FORMS:
Tablets: 50 mg, 100 mg

FLUTAMIDE
FLOO ta mide

TRADE NAME(S):
Eulexin

THERAPEUTIC CLASS:
Antiandrogen/ antineoplastic

GENERAL USES:
Prostate cancer

DOSAGE FORMS:
Capsules: 125 mg

FLUTICASONE (INHALED)
floo TIK a sone

TRADE NAME(S):
Flovent HFA, Flovent Rotadisk, Flovent Diskus

THERAPEUTIC CLASS:
Corticosteroid (inhaler)

GENERAL USES:
Asthma (chronic)

DOSAGE FORMS:
Aerosol: 44 mcg/ actuation, 110 mcg/ actuation, 220 mcg/ actuation; Inhaler: 50 mcg/actuation, 100 mcg/actuation, 250 mcg/actuation

FLUTICASONE (NASAL)
floo TIK a sone

TRADE NAME(S):
Flonase, Veramyst

THERAPEUTIC CLASS:
Corticosteroid (nasal)

GENERAL USES:
Allergies

DOSAGE FORMS:
Nasal spray: 50 mcg/
spray, 27.5 mcg/spray

FLUTICASONE PROPIONATE (TOPICAL)
floo TIK a sone
TRADE NAME(S):
Cutivate
THERAPEUTIC CLASS:
Corticosteroid (topical)
GENERAL USES:
Various skin conditions
DOSAGE FORMS:
Cream: 0.05%; Ointment:
0.005%

FLUTICASONE/ SALMETEROL
floo TIK a sone/sal ME te
role
TRADE NAME(S):
Advair Diskus
THERAPEUTIC CLASS:
Corticosteroid/
bronchodilator
GENERAL USES:
Asthma (chronic), COPD
DOSAGE FORMS:
Inhalation: 0.1 mg/
0.05 mg/inhalation,
0.25 mg/0.05 mg/
inhalation, 0.5 mg/
0.05 mg/inhalation

FLUVASTATIN
FLOO va sta tin

TRADE NAME(S):
Lescol, Lescol XL
THERAPEUTIC CLASS:
Antilipemic
GENERAL USES:
Hyperlipidemia,
secondary prevention of
CHD
DOSAGE FORMS:
Capsules: 20 mg, 40 mg;
Extended-release tablets:
80 mg

FLUVOXAMINE
floo VOKS a meen
TRADE NAME(S):
Luvox, Luvox CR
THERAPEUTIC CLASS:
Antidepressant
GENERAL USES:
OCD
DOSAGE FORMS:
Tablets: 25 mg, 50 mg,
100 mg; Extended-release
capsules: 100 mg, 150 mg

FOLIC ACID/ CYANOCOBALAMIN/ PYRIDOXINE
FOE lik AS id/sye an oh koe
BAL a min/peer i DOKS een
TRADE NAME(S):
Foltx
THERAPEUTIC CLASS:
Vitamin
GENERAL USES:
Nutritional
supplementation

DOSAGE FORMS:
Tablets: 2.5 mg/1 mg/
25 mg

**FONDAPARINUX
SODIUM**
fon da PARE i nuks
TRADE NAME(S):
Arixtra
THERAPEUTIC CLASS:
Anticoagulant (LMWH)
GENERAL USES:
Prevention of blood clots
DOSAGE FORMS:
Injection: 2.5 mg

FORMOTEROL
for MOE te rol
TRADE NAME(S):
Foradil
THERAPEUTIC CLASS:
Bronchodilator
GENERAL USES:
Asthma (chronic)
DOSAGE FORMS:
Inhalation: 12 mcg/
inhalation

**FORMOTEROL
FUMARATE**
for MOE te rol fue MAR ate
TRADE NAME(S):
Perforomist
THERAPEUTIC CLASS:
Bronchodilator
GENERAL USES:
COPD

DOSAGE FORMS:
Inhalation solution:
20 mcg/2 mL

FOSAMPRENAVIR
FOS am pren a veer
TRADE NAME(S):
Lexiva
THERAPEUTIC CLASS:
Antiviral
GENERAL USES:
HIV infection
DOSAGE FORMS:
Tablets: 700 mg; Oral
suspension: 50 mg/mL

**FOSAPREPITANT
DIMEGLUMINE**
FOS ap RE pi tant dye MEG
loo meen
TRADE NAME(S):
Emend
THERAPEUTIC CLASS:
Antiemetic
GENERAL USES:
Chemotherapy-induced
nausea/vomiting
DOSAGE FORMS:
Injection: 115 mg

FOSCARNET
fos KAR net
TRADE NAME(S):
Foscavir
THERAPEUTIC CLASS:
Antiviral
GENERAL USES:
CMV retinitis, herpes

simplex virus
infections

DOSAGE FORMS:
Injection: 12 g

FOSINOPRIL
foe SIN oh pril
TRADE NAME(S):
Monopril
THERAPEUTIC CLASS:
Antihypertensive, cardiac
agent
GENERAL USES:
Hypertension, heart failure
DOSAGE FORMS:
Tablets: 10 mg, 20 mg,
40 mg

FOSPHENYTOIN
FOS fen i toyn
TRADE NAME(S):
Cerebyx
THERAPEUTIC CLASS:
Anticonvulsants
GENERAL USES:
Seizures
DOSAGE FORMS:
Injection: 150 mg, 750 mg

FROVATRIPTAN
froe va TRIP tan
TRADE NAME(S):
Frova
THERAPEUTIC CLASS:
Antimigraine agent
GENERAL USES:
Acute treatment of

migraine
DOSAGE FORMS:
Tablets: 2.5 mg

FULVESTRANT
fool VES trant
TRADE NAME(S):
Faslodex
THERAPEUTIC CLASS:
Antineoplastic
GENERAL USES:
Breast cancer
DOSAGE FORMS:
Injection: 125 mg, 250 mg

FUROSEMIDE
fyoor OH se mide
TRADE NAME(S):
Lasix
THERAPEUTIC CLASS:
Diuretic
GENERAL USES:
CHF- and pulmonary-
related edema,
hypertension
DOSAGE FORMS:
Tablets: 20 mg, 40 mg,
80 mg; Solution:
10 mg/mL, 40 mg/5 mL;
Injection: 20 mg, 40 mg,
100 mg

GABAPENTIN
GA ba pen tin
TRADE NAME(S):
Neurontin

THERAPEUTIC CLASS:
Anticonvulsant

GENERAL USES:
Seizures, postherpetic neuralgia

DOSAGE FORMS:
Capsules: 100 mg, 300 mg, 400 mg; Tablets: 100 mg, 300 mg, 400 mg, 600 mg, 800 mg; Solution: 250 mg/ 5 mL

GADOBENATE DIMEGLUMINE
gad oh BEN ate dye MEG loo meen

TRADE NAME(S):
Multihance

THERAPEUTIC CLASS:
Radiopaque agent

GENERAL USES:
Enhancement of MRI

DOSAGE FORMS:
Injection: 2.645 g, 5.290 g, 7.935 g, 10.58 g, 26.45 g, 52.9 g

GADOXETATE DISODIUM
ga DOKS e tate

TRADE NAME(S):
Eovist

THERAPEUTIC CLASS:
Radiopaque agent

GENERAL USES:
MRI of liver

DOSAGE FORMS:
Injection: 10 mL

GALANTAMINE
ga LAN ta meen

TRADE NAME(S):
Razadyne ER, Razadyne

THERAPEUTIC CLASS:
Alzheimer's agent

GENERAL USES:
Mild to moderate dementia of Alzheimer's

DOSAGE FORMS:
Tablets: 4 mg, 8 mg, 12 mg; Solution: 4 mg/ mL; Extended-release capsules: 8 mg, 16 mg, 24 mg

GALSULFASE
gal SUL fase

TRADE NAME(S):
Naglazyme

THERAPEUTIC CLASS:
Enzyme

GENERAL USES:
Mucopolysaccharidosis VI

DOSAGE FORMS:
Injection: 5 mg

GANCICLOVIR
gan SYE kloe veer

TRADE NAME(S):
Cytovene

THERAPEUTIC CLASS:
Antiviral

GENERAL USES:
CMV retinitis and infection

DOSAGE FORMS:
Capsules: 250 mg,
500 mg; Injection:
500 mg

GATIFLOXACIN (OCULAR)
ga ti FLOKS a sin
TRADE NAME(S):
Zymar
THERAPEUTIC CLASS:
Anti-infective
GENERAL USES:
Ocular infections
DOSAGE FORMS:
Ophthalmic solution:
0.3%

GEFITINIB
ge FI tye nib
TRADE NAME(S):
Iressa
THERAPEUTIC CLASS:
Antineoplastic
GENERAL USES:
Non-small-cell lung
cancer
DOSAGE FORMS:
Tablets: 250 mg

GEMFIBROZIL
jem FI broe zil
TRADE NAME(S):
Lopid
THERAPEUTIC CLASS:
Antilipemic

GENERAL USES:
Hyperlipidemia
DOSAGE FORMS:
Tablets: 600 mg

GEMIFLOXACIN
je mi FLOKS a sin
TRADE NAME(S):
Factive
THERAPEUTIC CLASS:
Anti-infective
GENERAL USES:
Bacterial infections
DOSAGE FORMS:
Tablets: 320 mg

GEMTUZUMAB OZOGAMICIN
gem TOO zoo mab oh zog a
MY sin
TRADE NAME(S):
Mylotarg
THERAPEUTIC CLASS:
Antineoplastic
GENERAL USES:
Acute myeloid
leukemia
DOSAGE FORMS:
Injection: 5 mg

GENTAMICIN
jen ta MYE sin
TRADE NAME(S):
Garamycin, Genoptic,
Gentak
THERAPEUTIC CLASS:
Ocular agent (anti-
infective)

GENERAL USES:
Ocular infections

DOSAGE FORMS:
Ophthalmic ointment:
3 mg/g; Ophthalmic
solution: 3 mg/mL

GENTAMICIN (INJECTION)
jen ta MYE sin

TRADE NAME(S):
Garamycin

THERAPEUTIC CLASS:
Anti-infective

GENERAL USES:
Bacterial infections

DOSAGE FORMS:
Injection: 20 mg,
60 mg, 80 mg,
800 mg

GLIMEPIRIDE
GLYE me pye ride

TRADE NAME(S):
Amaryl

THERAPEUTIC CLASS:
Antidiabetic

GENERAL USES:
Diabetes (type 2)

DOSAGE FORMS:
Tablets: 1 mg, 2 mg, 4 mg

GLIPIZIDE
GLIP i zide

TRADE NAME(S):
Glucotrol,
Glucotrol XL

THERAPEUTIC CLASS:
Antidiabetic

GENERAL USES:
Diabetes (type 2)

DOSAGE FORMS:
Tablets: 5 mg, 10 mg;
Extended-release tablets:
2.5 mg, 5 mg, 10 mg

GLYBURIDE
GLYE byoor ide

TRADE NAME(S):
Diabeta, Micronase,
Glynase

THERAPEUTIC CLASS:
Antidiabetic

GENERAL USES:
Diabetes (type 2)

DOSAGE FORMS:
Tablets: 1.25 mg, 2.5 mg,
5 mg; Micronized tablets:
1.5 mg, 3 mg, 4.5 mg,
6 mg

GLYBURIDE/ METFORMIN
GLYE byoor ide/met FOR min

TRADE NAME(S):
Glucovance

THERAPEUTIC CLASS:
Antidiabetic

GENERAL USES:
Diabetes (type 2)

DOSAGE FORMS:
Tablets: 1.25 mg/250 mg,
2.5 mg/500 mg, 5 mg/
500 mg

GRANISETRON
gra NI se tron
TRADE NAME(S):
Kytril
THERAPEUTIC CLASS:
Antiemetic
GENERAL USES:
Postoperative
chemotherapy nausea/
vomiting
DOSAGE FORMS:
Tablets: 1 mg; Injection:
1 mg, 4 mg; Oral solution:
2 mg/10 mL

**GRISEOFULVIN
MICROSIZE**
gri see oh FUL vin
TRADE NAME(S):
Fulvicin, Grifulvin
THERAPEUTIC CLASS:
Antifungal
GENERAL USES:
Fungal infections
DOSAGE FORMS:
Tablets: 250 mg, 500 mg;
Capsules: 125 mg,
250 mg; Suspension:
125 mg/5 mL

**GRISEOFULVIN
ULTRAMICROSIZE**
gri see oh FUL vin
TRADE NAME(S):
Fulvicin P/G, Grisactin,
Gris-PEG
THERAPEUTIC CLASS:
Antifungal

GENERAL USES:
Fungal infections
DOSAGE FORMS:
Tablets: 125 mg, 165 mg,
250 mg, 330 mg

**GUAIFENESIN/
PSEUDOEPHEDRINE**
gwye FEN e sin/soo doe e
FED rin
TRADE NAME(S):
Guaifenex PSE
THERAPEUTIC CLASS:
Mucolytic/decongestant
GENERAL USES:
Cough and colds
DOSAGE FORMS:
Sustained-release tablets:
600 mg/60 mg,
600 mg/120 mg,
1200 mg/60 mg,
1200 mg/120 mg

GUANABENZ
GWAHN a benz
TRADE NAME(S):
Wytensin
THERAPEUTIC CLASS:
Antihypertensive
GENERAL USES:
Hypertension
DOSAGE FORMS:
Tablets: 4 mg, 8 mg

GUANADREL
GWAHN a drel
TRADE NAME(S):
Hylorel

Therapeutic Class:
Antihypertensive
General Uses:
Hypertension
Dosage Forms:
Tablets: 10 mg,
25 mg

GUANETHIDINE
gwahn ETH i deen
Trade Name(s):
Ismelin
Therapeutic Class:
Antihypertensive
General Uses:
Hypertension
Dosage Forms:
Tablets: 10 mg, 25 mg

GUANFACINE
GWAHN fa seen
Trade Name(s):
Tenex
Therapeutic Class:
Antihypertensive
General Uses:
Hypertension
Dosage Forms:
Tablets: 1 mg, 2 mg

HALCINONIDE
hal SIN oh nide
Trade Name(s):
Halog, Halog-E
Therapeutic Class:
Corticosteroid
(topical)

General Uses:
Various skin conditions
Dosage Forms:
Ointment, Solution, and
Cream: 0.1%; Cream:
0.025%

HALOFANTRINE
ha loe FAN trin
Trade Name(s):
Halfan
Therapeutic Class:
Antimalarial
General Uses:
Malaria treatment
Dosage Forms:
Tablets: 250 mg

HALOPERIDOL
ha loe PER i dole
Trade Name(s):
Haldol
Therapeutic Class:
Antipsychotic
General Uses:
Psychotic/behavioral
disorders, Tourette's
Dosage Forms:
Tablets: 0.5 mg, 1 mg,
2 mg, 5 mg, 10 mg,
20 mg; Concentrated
solution: 2 mg/mL;
Injection: 5 mg, 50 mg,
100 mg, 250 mg, 500 mg

HALOPROGIN
ha loe PROE jin

TRADE NAME(S):
  Halotex
THERAPEUTIC CLASS:
  Antifungal (topical)
GENERAL USES:
  Athlete's foot, jock itch,
  ringworm, tinea versicolor
DOSAGE FORMS:
  Cream and Solution: 1%

HEPARIN
HEP a rin
TRADE NAME(S):
  Heparin
THERAPEUTIC CLASS:
  Anticoagulant
GENERAL USES:
  Prevention of blood clots
DOSAGE FORMS:
  Various concentrations

HETASTARCH
HET a starch
TRADE NAME(S):
  Hespan
THERAPEUTIC CLASS:
  Plasma expander
GENERAL USES:
  Shock
DOSAGE FORMS:
  Injection: 30 g

HUMAN PAPILLOMAVIRUS (HPV) VACCINE
pap i LOE ma VYE rus vak
SEEN

TRADE NAME(S):
  Gardasil
THERAPEUTIC CLASS:
  Vaccine
GENERAL USES:
  Prevention of HPV in
  females
DOSAGE FORMS:
  Injection: 0.5 mL (various
  HPV proteins)

HYALURONIDASE
hye al yoor ON i dase
TRADE NAME(S):
  Hydase, Amphadase
THERAPEUTIC CLASS:
  Enzyme
GENERAL USES:
  Increase absorption
  and dispersion of
  drugs
DOSAGE FORMS:
  Injection: 150 units,
  300 units

HYALURONIDASE (OVINE)
hye al yoor ON i dase
TRADE NAME(S):
  Vitrase
THERAPEUTIC CLASS:
  Enzyme
GENERAL USES:
  Increase absorption of
  injected drugs
DOSAGE FORMS:
  Injection: 6200 units

HYDRALAZINE

hye DRAL a zeen

Trade Name(s):
Apresoline

Therapeutic Class:
Antihypertensive

General Uses:
Hypertension

Dosage Forms:
Tablets: 10 mg, 25 mg,
50 mg, 100 mg; Injection:
20 mg

HYDRALAZINE/HCTZ

hye DRAL a zeen/hye droe
klor oh THYE a zide

Trade Name(s):
Apresazide

Therapeutic Class:
Antihypertensive/diuretic

General Uses:
Hypertension

Dosage Forms:
Tablets: 25 mg/25 mg,
50 mg/50 mg, 100 mg/
50 mg

HYDRALAZINE/ ISOSORBIDE DINITRATE

hye DRAL a zeen/eye soe
SOR bide dye NYE trate

Trade Name(s):
BiDil

Therapeutic Class:
Antihypertensive/
Antianginal

General Uses:
Heart failure

Dosage Forms:
Tablets: 37.5 mg/20 mg

HYDROCHLORO- THIAZIDE

hye droe klor oh THYE a zide

Trade Name(s):
Esidrix, HydroDIURIL,
Oretic

Therapeutic Class:
Diuretic

General Uses:
CHF-related edema,
hypertension

Dosage Forms:
Tablets: 25 mg, 50 mg,
100 mg; Capsules:
12.5 mg; Solution:
50 mg/5 mL

HYDROCODONE/ CHLORPHENIRAMINE

hye droe KOE done/klor fen
IR a meen

Trade Name(s):
Tussionex
Pennkinetic

Therapeutic Class:
Analgesic/Antihistamine

General Uses:
Cough and cold

Dosage Forms:
Extended-release
suspension: 10 mg/8 mg
per 5 mL

HYDROCORTISONE (ORAL)

hye droe KOR ti sone

TRADE NAME(S):
Cortef

THERAPEUTIC CLASS:
Glucocorticoid

GENERAL USES:
Endocrine, skin, blood disorders

DOSAGE FORMS:
Tablets: 5 mg, 10 mg, 20 mg

HYDROCORTISONE (TOPICAL)

hye droe KOR ti sone

TRADE NAME(S):
Hycort, Cort-Dome, Dermacort, many others

THERAPEUTIC CLASS:
Corticosteroid (topical)

GENERAL USES:
Various skin conditions

DOSAGE FORMS:
Ointment, Lotion, and Cream: 0.5%, 1%, 2.5%; Lotion: 2%; Gel, Solution, and Spray: 1%

HYDROCORTISONE ACETATE

hye droe KOR ti sone

TRADE NAME(S):
Hydrocortone Acetate

THERAPEUTIC CLASS:
Glucocorticoid

GENERAL USES:
Endocrine, skin, blood disorders

DOSAGE FORMS:
Injection: 125 mg, 250 mg, 500 mg

HYDROCORTISONE SODIUM SUCCINATE

hye droe KOR ti sone

TRADE NAME(S):
Solu-Cortef, A-Hydrocort

THERAPEUTIC CLASS:
Glucocorticoid

GENERAL USES:
Endocrine, skin, blood disorders

DOSAGE FORMS:
Injection: 100 mg, 250 mg, 500 mg, 1000 mg

HYDROXY-AMPHETAMINE

hye droks ee am FET a meen

TRADE NAME(S):
Paredrine

THERAPEUTIC CLASS:
Ocular agent

GENERAL USES:
Pupil dilation

DOSAGE FORMS:
Ophthalmic solution: 1%

HYDROXY-CHLOROQUINE

hye droks ee KLOR oh kwin

TRADE NAME(S):
Plaquenil

THERAPEUTIC CLASS:
Antirheumatic agent

GENERAL USES:
Rheumatoid arthritis, systemic lupus erythematosus

DOSAGE FORMS:
Tablets: 200 mg

HYDROXYZINE

hye DROKS i zeen

TRADE NAME(S):
Atarax, Vistaril

THERAPEUTIC CLASS:
Antihistamine

GENERAL USES:
Itching, sedation

DOSAGE FORMS:
Tablets: 10 mg, 25 mg, 50 mg, 100 mg; Capsules: 25 mg, 50 mg, 100 mg; Syrup: 10 mg/5 mL; Suspension: 25 mg/5 mL; Injection: 25 mg, 50 mg

IBANDRONATE

eye BAN droh nate

TRADE NAME(S):
Boniva

THERAPEUTIC CLASS:
Bisphosphonate

GENERAL USES:
Postmenopausal osteoporosis

DOSAGE FORMS:
Injection: 3 mg; Tablets: 2.5 mg, 150 mg

IBRITUMOMAB

ib ri TYOO mo mab

TRADE NAME(S):
Zevalin

THERAPEUTIC CLASS:
Monoclonal antibody

GENERAL USES:
Non-Hodgkin's lymphoma

DOSAGE FORMS:
Injection: 3.2 mg

IBUPROFEN

eye byoo PROE fen

TRADE NAME(S):
Motrin, Advil, Nuprin, many others

THERAPEUTIC CLASS:
Analgesic, antipyretic, anti-inflammatory

GENERAL USES:
Pain, fever, arthritis

DOSAGE FORMS:
Tablets: 100 mg, 200 mg, 300 mg, 400 mg, 600 mg, 800 mg; Chewable tablets: 50 mg, 100 mg; Capsules: 200 mg; Liquid or Suspension: 100 mg/5 mL; Suspension: 100 mg/2.5 mL; Drops: 40 mg/mL

IDOXURIDINE
eye doks YOOR i deen
TRADE NAME(S):
　Herplex
THERAPEUTIC CLASS:
　Ocular agent (antiviral)
GENERAL USES:
　Ocular herpes
　infections
DOSAGE FORMS:
　Ophthalmic solution: 0.1%

IDURSULFASE
eye dur SUL fase
TRADE NAME(S):
　Elaprase
THERAPEUTIC CLASS:
　Enzyme
GENERAL USES:
　Hunter syndrome
DOSAGE FORMS:
　Injection: 5 mL

ILOPROST
EYE loe prost
TRADE NAME(S):
　Ventavis
THERAPEUTIC CLASS:
　Antihypertensive
GENERAL USES:
　Pulmonary hypertension
DOSAGE FORMS:
　Inhalation: 10 mcg,
　20 mcg

IMATINIB
eye MAT eh nib

TRADE NAME(S):
　Gleevec
THERAPEUTIC CLASS:
　Antineoplastic
GENERAL USES:
　Chronic myeloid leukemia,
　GI stromal tumors
DOSAGE FORMS:
　Capsules: 100 mg

IMIPENEM/CILASTATIN
i mi PEN em/sye la STAT in
TRADE NAME(S):
　Primaxin
THERAPEUTIC CLASS:
　Anti-infective
GENERAL USES:
　Bacterial infections
DOSAGE FORMS:
　Injection: 250 mg/
　250 mg, 500 mg/500 mg,
　750 mg/750 mg

IMIPRAMINE HCL
im IP ra meen
TRADE NAME(S):
　Tofranil
THERAPEUTIC CLASS:
　Antidepressant
GENERAL USES:
　Depression,
　childhood
　bedwetting
DOSAGE FORMS:
　Tablets: 10 mg, 25 mg,
　50 mg

IMIPRAMINE PAMOATE
im IP ra meen
Trade Name(s):
Tofranil-PM
Therapeutic Class:
Antidepressant
General Uses:
Depression
Dosage Forms:
Capsules: 75 mg, 100 mg,
125 mg, 150 mg

IMIQUIMOD
i mi KWI mod
Trade Name(s):
Aldara
Therapeutic Class:
Immunomodulator
(topical)
General Uses:
Actinic keratosis, genital
and anal warts, basal cell
carcinoma
Dosage Forms:
Cream: 5%

INDAPAMIDE
in DAP a mide
Trade Name(s):
Lozol
Therapeutic Class:
Diuretic
General Uses:
CHF, hypertension
Dosage Forms:
Tablets: 1.25 mg, 2.5 mg

INDINAVIR
in DIN a veer
Trade Name(s):
Crixivan
Therapeutic Class:
Antiviral
General Uses:
HIV infection
Dosage Forms:
Capsules: 100 mg,
200 mg, 333 mg, 400 mg

INDOMETHACIN
in doe METH a sin
Trade Name(s):
Indocin, Indocin ER,
Indocin SR
Therapeutic Class:
Anti-inflammatory/
analgesic
General Uses:
Various arthritis
conditions, pain
Dosage Forms:
Capsules: 25 mg,
50 mg; Sustained-
release capsules: 75 mg;
Suspension: 25 mg/5 mL

INFLIXIMAB
in FLIKS i mab
Trade Name(s):
Remicade
Therapeutic Class:
Monoclonal antibody
General Uses:
Crohn's disease, various

arthritis syndromes,
ulcerative colitis,
psoriasis, psoriatic
arthritis
DOSAGE FORMS:
Injection: 100 mg

**INFLUENZA VIRUS
VACCINE, LIVE
(INTRANASAL)**
in floo EN za VYE rus vak
SEEN
TRADE NAME(S):
FluMist
THERAPEUTIC CLASS:
Vaccine
GENERAL USES:
Prevention of influenza
DOSAGE FORMS:
Nasal spray: 0.5 mL

INSULIN, ASPART
IN su lin AS part
TRADE NAME(S):
NovoLog
THERAPEUTIC CLASS:
Antidiabetic
GENERAL USES:
Diabetes
DOSAGE FORMS:
Injection: 100 units/mL

INSULIN, DETEMIR
IN su lin DE te mir
TRADE NAME(S):
Levemir
THERAPEUTIC CLASS:
Antidiabetic

GENERAL USES:
Diabetes
DOSAGE FORMS:
100 units/mL

INSULIN, GLARGINE
IN su lin GLAR jeen
TRADE NAME(S):
Lantus
THERAPEUTIC CLASS:
Antidiabetic
GENERAL USES:
Diabetes
DOSAGE FORMS:
Injection: 100 units/mL

INSULIN, GLULISINE
IN su lin gloo LIS een
TRADE NAME(S):
Apidra
THERAPEUTIC CLASS:
Antidiabetic
GENERAL USES:
Diabetes
DOSAGE FORMS:
Injection: 100 units/mL

**INSULIN, HUMAN
(rDNA)**
IN su lin
TRADE NAME(S):
Exubera
THERAPEUTIC CLASS:
Antidiabetic
GENERAL USES:
Diabetes
DOSAGE FORMS:
Oral inhalation: 1 mg, 3 mg

INSULIN, ISOPHANE SUSPENSION

IN su lin EYE soe fane

Trade Name(s):
Novolin N, Humulin N

Therapeutic Class:
Antidiabetic

General Uses:
Diabetes

Dosage Forms:
Injection: 100 units/mL

INSULIN, ISOPHANE SUSPENSION AND INSULIN REGULAR

IN su lin

Trade Name(s):
Humulin 50/50, Novolin 70/30, Humulin 70/30

Therapeutic Class:
Antidiabetic

General Uses:
Diabetes

Dosage Forms:
Injection: 100 units/mL

INSULIN, LISPRO

IN su lin LYE sproe

Trade Name(s):
Humalog

Therapeutic Class:
Antidiabetic

General Uses:
Diabetes

Dosage Forms:
Injection: 100 units/mL

INSULIN, LISPRO PROTAMINE SUSPENSION AND INSULIN LISPRO

IN su lin

Trade Name(s):
Humalog 75/25

Therapeutic Class:
Antidiabetic

General Uses:
Diabetes

Dosage Forms:
Injection: 100 units/mL

INSULIN, REGULAR

IN su lin

Trade Name(s):
Novolin R, Humulin R

Therapeutic Class:
Antidiabetic

General Uses:
Diabetes

Dosage Forms:
Injection: 100 units/mL

INSULIN, ZINC SUSPENSION

IN su lin

Trade Name(s):
Humulin L

Therapeutic Class:
Antidiabetic

General Uses:
Diabetes

Dosage Forms:
Injection: 100 units/mL

INSULIN, ZINC SUSPENSION, EXTENDED

IN su lin

TRADE NAME(S):
Humulin U

THERAPEUTIC CLASS:
Antidiabetic

GENERAL USES:
Diabetes

DOSAGE FORMS:
Injection: 100 units/mL

INTERFERON ALFA-2a

in ter FEER on

TRADE NAME(S):
Roferon-A

THERAPEUTIC CLASS:
Immune modulator

GENERAL USES:
Leukemia, AIDS sarcoma

DOSAGE FORMS:
Injection: 3 million international units, 6 million international units, 9 million international units, 18 million international units, 36 million international units

INTERFERON ALFA-2b

in ter FEER on

TRADE NAME(S):
Intron-A

THERAPEUTIC CLASS:
Immune modulator

GENERAL USES:
Leukemia, AIDS sarcoma, hepatitis B, C (chronic)

DOSAGE FORMS:
Injection: 3 million international units, 5 million international units, 10 million international units, 18 million international units, 25 million international units, 50 million international units

INTERFERON BETA-1a

in ter FEER on

TRADE NAME(S):
Avonex, Rebif

THERAPEUTIC CLASS:
Immune modulator

GENERAL USES:
Multiple sclerosis

DOSAGE FORMS:
Injection: 6.6 million international units (33 mcg)

INTERFERON BETA-1b

in ter FEER on

TRADE NAME(S):
Betaseron

THERAPEUTIC CLASS:
Immune modulator

GENERAL USES:
Multiple sclerosis

DOSAGE FORMS:
Injection: 9.6 million

international units
(0.3 mg)

IODOQUINOL
eye oh doe KWIN ole
TRADE NAME(S):
Yodoxin
THERAPEUTIC CLASS:
Antituberculosis agent
GENERAL USES:
Tuberculosis
DOSAGE FORMS:
Tablets: 210 mg, 650 mg;
Powder: 25 g

IPRATROPIUM
i pra TROE pee um
TRADE NAME(S):
Atrovent
THERAPEUTIC CLASS:
Bronchodilator
GENERAL USES:
Bronchospasm,
asthma
DOSAGE FORMS:
Inhalation solution:
0.02%; Inhaler: 18 mcg/
inhalation; Nasal spray:
0.03%, 0.06%

IPRATROPIUM/
ALBUTEROL
i pra TROE pee um/al BYOO
ter ole
TRADE NAME(S):
Combivent
THERAPEUTIC CLASS:
Bronchodilator

GENERAL USES:
Bronchospasm
DOSAGE FORMS:
Inhaler: 18 mcg/103 mcg/
inhalation

IRBESARTAN
ir be SAR tan
TRADE NAME(S):
Avapro
THERAPEUTIC CLASS:
Antihypertensive
GENERAL USES:
Hypertension, diabetic
nephropathy
DOSAGE FORMS:
Tablets: 75 mg, 150 mg,
300 mg

IRBESARTAN/HCTZ
ir be SAR tan/hye droe klor
oh THYE a zide
TRADE NAME(S):
Avalide
THERAPEUTIC CLASS:
Antihypertensive/
diuretic
GENERAL USES:
Hypertension
DOSAGE FORMS:
Tablets: 150 mg/12.5 mg,
300 mg/12.5 mg

ISOCARBOXAZID
eye so kar BOKS a zid
TRADE NAME(S):
Marplan

THERAPEUTIC CLASS:
Antidepressant
GENERAL USES:
Depression
DOSAGE FORMS:
Tablets: 10 mg

ISOETHARINE
eye soe ETH a reen
TRADE NAME(S):
Bronkosol
THERAPEUTIC CLASS:
Bronchodilator
GENERAL USES:
Bronchospasm,
asthma
DOSAGE FORMS:
Inhalation solution: 1%

ISONIAZID
eye soe NYE a zid
TRADE NAME(S):
Laniazid, Nydrazid
THERAPEUTIC CLASS:
Antituberculosis
agent
GENERAL USES:
Tuberculosis
DOSAGE FORMS:
Tablets: 50 mg, 100 mg,
300 mg; Syrup: 50 mg/
5 mL; Injection: 1 g

ISOPROTERENOL
eye soe proe TER e nole
TRADE NAME(S):
Isuprel, Medihaler

THERAPEUTIC CLASS:
Bronchodilator
GENERAL USES:
Bronchospasm,
asthma
DOSAGE FORMS:
Inhalation solution: 0.5%,
1%; Inhaler: 103 mcg/
inhalation, 80 mcg/
inhalation

ISOSORBIDE DINITRATE
eye soe SOR bide dye NYE
trate
TRADE NAME(S):
Isordil, Sorbitrate
THERAPEUTIC CLASS:
Antianginal
GENERAL USES:
Angina
DOSAGE FORMS:
Tablets: 5 mg, 10 mg,
20 mg, 30 mg, 40 mg;
Sustained-release tablets
and capsules: 40 mg;
Sublingual tablets:
2.5 mg, 5 mg, 10 mg;
Chewable tablets: 5 mg,
10 mg

ISOSORBIDE MONONITRATE
eye soe SOR bide mon oh
NYE trate
TRADE NAME(S):
Ismo, Monoket,
Imdur

THERAPEUTIC CLASS:
Antianginal
GENERAL USES:
Angina
DOSAGE FORMS:
Tablets: 10 mg, 20 mg;
Extended-release tablets:
30 mg, 60 mg, 120 mg

ISOTRETINOIN
eye soe TRET i noyn
TRADE NAME(S):
Accutane
THERAPEUTIC CLASS:
Retinoid
GENERAL USES:
Severe cystic acne
DOSAGE FORMS:
Capsules: 10 mg, 20 mg,
40 mg

ISRADIPINE
iz RA di peen
TRADE NAME(S):
DynaCirc CR,
DynaCirc
THERAPEUTIC CLASS:
Antihypertensive
GENERAL USES:
Hypertension
DOSAGE FORMS:
Capsules: 2.5 mg, 5 mg;
Controlled-release tablets:
5 mg, 10 mg

ITRACONAZOLE
i tra KOE na zole

TRADE NAME(S):
Sporanox
THERAPEUTIC CLASS:
Antifungal
GENERAL USES:
Fungal infections
DOSAGE FORMS:
Capsules: 100 mg;
Solution: 10 mg/mL;
Injection: 10 mg

IXABEPILONE
iks ab EP i lone
TRADE NAME(S):
Ixempra
THERAPEUTIC CLASS:
Antineoplastic
GENERAL USES:
Breast cancer
DOSAGE FORMS:
Injection: 15 mg,
45 mg

KANAMYCIN
kan a MYE sin
TRADE NAME(S):
Kantrex
THERAPEUTIC CLASS:
Anti-infective
GENERAL USES:
Bacterial infections
DOSAGE FORMS:
Injection: 150 mg, 1 g,
2 g, 3 g

KETOCONAZOLE
kee toe KOE na zole

TRADE NAME(S):
Nizoral, Xolegel
THERAPEUTIC CLASS:
Antifungal (oral and topical)
GENERAL USES:
Fungal infections
DOSAGE FORMS:
Tablets: 200 mg; Shampoo, Gel, and Cream: 2%

KETOPROFEN
kee toe PROE fen
TRADE NAME(S):
Orudis KT, Actron, Orudis, Oruvail
THERAPEUTIC CLASS:
Anti-inflammatory/ analgesic
GENERAL USES:
Osteoarthritis, rheumatoid arthritis, pain
DOSAGE FORMS:
Capsules: 12.5 mg, 25 mg, 50 mg, 75 mg; Extended-release capsules: 100 mg, 150 mg, 200 mg

KETOROLAC
kee toe ROLE ak
TRADE NAME(S):
Toradol
THERAPEUTIC CLASS:
Anti-inflammatory/ analgesic
GENERAL USES:
Severe acute pain (short-term therapy)
DOSAGE FORMS:
Tablets: 10 mg; Injection: 15 mg, 30 mg, 60 mg

KETOROLAC (OCULAR)
kee toe ROLE ak
TRADE NAME(S):
Acular
THERAPEUTIC CLASS:
Ocular agent
GENERAL USES:
Allergic conjunctivitis
DOSAGE FORMS:
Ophthalmic solution: 0.5%

KETOTIFEN
kee toe TYE fen
TRADE NAME(S):
Zaditor
THERAPEUTIC CLASS:
Ocular agent
GENERAL USES:
Allergic conjunctivitis
DOSAGE FORMS:
Ophthalmic solution: 0.025%

LABETALOL
la BET a lole
TRADE NAME(S):
Normodyne, Trandate

Therapeutic Class:
Antihypertensive
General Uses:
Hypertension
Dosage Forms:
Tablets: 100 mg, 200 mg,
300 mg

LAMIVUDINE (3TC)
la MI vyoo deen
Trade Name(s):
Epivir, Epivir-HBV
Therapeutic Class:
Antiviral
General Uses:
HIV infection
Dosage Forms:
Tablets: 100 mg, 150 mg;
Solution: 5 mg/mL,
10 mg/mL

LAMIVUDINE/ ZIDOVUDINE
la MI vyoo deen/zye DOE
vyoo deen
Trade Name(s):
Combivir
Therapeutic Class:
Antiviral
General Uses:
HIV infection
Dosage Forms:
Tablets: 150 mg/300 mg

LAMOTRIGINE
la MOE tri jeen
Trade Name(s):
Lamictal

Therapeutic Class:
Anticonvulsant
General Uses:
Seizures, bipolar disorder
Dosage Forms:
Tablets: 25 mg, 100 mg,
150 mg, 200 mg;
Chewable tablets: 5 mg,
25 mg

LANREOTIDE
lan REE oh tide
Trade Name(s):
Somatuline Depot
Therapeutic Class:
Hormone
General Uses:
Acromegaly
Dosage Forms:
Injection: 60 mg, 90 mg,
120 mg

LANSOPRAZOLE
lan SOE pra zole
Trade Name(s):
Prevacid
Therapeutic Class:
Gastric acid secretion
inhibitor
General Uses:
Duodenal ulcer,
GERD
Dosage Forms:
Delayed-release capsules
and suspension: 15 mg,
30 mg

LANSOPRAZOLE/ NAPROXEN
lan SOE pra zole/na PROKS en
Trade Name(s):
Prevacid/NapraPAC
Therapeutic Class:
Gastric acid secretion inhibitor/NSAID
General Uses:
Arthritis in patients at risk for gastric ulcers
Dosage Forms:
Tablets: 15 mg/375 mg, 15 mg/500 mg

LANTHANUM CARBONATE
LAN tha num
Trade Name(s):
Fosrenol
Therapeutic Class:
Phosphate binder
General Uses:
End-stage renal disease
Dosage Forms:
Tablets: 250 mg, 500 mg, 750 mg, 1000 mg

LAPATINIB
la PA ti nib
Trade Name(s):
Tykerb
Therapeutic Class:
Antineoplastic
General Uses:
Breast cancer
Dosage Forms:
Tablets: 250 mg

LARONIDASE
lair OH ni days
Trade Name(s):
Aldurazyme
Therapeutic Class:
Enzyme
General Uses:
Mucopolysaccharidosis I
Dosage Forms:
Injection: 2.9 mg

LATANOPROST
la TA noe prost
Trade Name(s):
Xalatan
Therapeutic Class:
Ocular agent
General Uses:
Glaucoma/ocular hypertension
Dosage Forms:
Ophthalmic solution: 0.005%

LEFLUNOMIDE
le FLOO noh mide
Trade Name(s):
Arava
Therapeutic Class:
Antirheumatic
General Uses:
Rheumatoid arthritis
Dosage Forms:
Tablets: 10 mg, 20 mg, 100 mg

LENALIDOMIDE
le na LID oh mide
TRADE NAME(S):
Revlimid
THERAPEUTIC CLASS:
Immunologic agent
GENERAL USES:
Myelodysplastic
syndrome
DOSAGE FORMS:
Capsules: 5 mg, 10 mg

LEPIRUDIN
le PEER u din
TRADE NAME(S):
Refludan
THERAPEUTIC CLASS:
Anticoagulant
GENERAL USES:
Heparin-induced
thrombocytopenia
DOSAGE FORMS:
Injection: 50 mg

LETROZOLE
LET roe zole
TRADE NAME(S):
Femara
THERAPEUTIC CLASS:
Antineoplastic
GENERAL USES:
Breast cancer
DOSAGE FORMS:
Tablets: 2.5 mg

LEVALBUTEROL
lev al BYOO ter ol

TRADE NAME(S):
Xopenox, Xopenox HFA
THERAPEUTIC CLASS:
Bronchodilator
GENERAL USES:
Bronchospasm
DOSAGE FORMS:
Solution for inhalation:
0.31 mg/3 mL, 0.63 mg/
3 mL, 1.25 mg/3 mL;
Oral aerosol: 45 mcg/
actuation; Concentrate:
1.25 mg/0.5 mL

LEVETIRACETAM
lee ve tye RA se tam
TRADE NAME(S):
Keppra, Keppra IV
THERAPEUTIC CLASS:
Anticonvulsant
GENERAL USES:
Partial seizures
DOSAGE FORMS:
Tablets: 250 mg, 500 mg,
750 mg, 1000 mg; Oral
solution: 100 mg/mL;
Injection: 500 mg

LEVOBETAXOLOL
lee voe be TAKS oh lol
TRADE NAME(S):
Betaxon
THERAPEUTIC CLASS:
Ocular agent
GENERAL USES:
Open-angle
glaucoma, ocular

DOSAGE FORMS:
Injection: 0.5 mg

LIDOCAINE (TRANSDERMAL)
LYE doe kane
TRADE NAME(S):
Lidoderm
THERAPEUTIC CLASS:
Anesthetic, local
GENERAL USES:
Postherpetic neuralgia
DOSAGE FORMS:
Patch: 5%

LIDOCAINE/ TETRACAINE
LYE doe kane/TET ra kane
TRADE NAME(S):
Synera
THERAPEUTIC CLASS:
Anesthetic
GENERAL USES:
Topical anesthesia
DOSAGE FORMS:
Patch: 70 mg/70 mg

LINDANE
LIN dane
TRADE NAME(S):
Kwell, G-well
THERAPEUTIC CLASS:
Scabicide/pediculicide (topical)
GENERAL USES:
Scabies, head lice

DOSAGE FORMS:
Lotion and Shampoo: 1%

LINEZOLID
li NE zoh lid
TRADE NAME(S):
Zyvox
THERAPEUTIC CLASS:
Anti-infective
GENERAL USES:
Vancomycin-resistant bacterial infections
DOSAGE FORMS:
Tablets: 400 mg, 600 mg; Suspension: 100 mg/ 5 mL; Injection: 200 mg, 400 mg, 600 mg

LIOTHYRONINE
lye oh THYE roe neen
TRADE NAME(S):
Cytomel, Triostat
THERAPEUTIC CLASS:
Hormone (thyroid)
GENERAL USES:
Hypothyroidism
DOSAGE FORMS:
Tablets: 5 mcg, 25 mcg, 50 mcg; Injection: 10 mcg

LISDEXAMFETAMINE DIMESYLATE
lis DEX am FET a meen dye MES i late
TRADE NAME(S):
Vyvanse

THERAPEUTIC CLASS:
  Amphetamine
GENERAL USES:
  ADHD
DOSAGE FORMS:
  Capsules: 20 mg, 30 mg,
  40 mg, 50 mg, 60 mg,
  70 mg

LISINOPRIL
lyse IN oh pril
TRADE NAME(S):
  Zestril, Prinivil
THERAPEUTIC CLASS:
  Antihypertensive, cardiac
  agent
GENERAL USES:
  Hypertension, heart
  failure, MI
DOSAGE FORMS:
  Tablets: 2.5 mg, 5 mg,
  10 mg, 20 mg, 40 mg

LISINOPRIL/HCTZ
lyse IN oh pril/hye droe klor
oh THYE a zide
TRADE NAME(S):
  Zestoretic, Prinzide
THERAPEUTIC CLASS:
  Antihypertensive/diuretic
GENERAL USES:
  Hypertension
DOSAGE FORMS:
  Tablets: 10 mg/12.5 mg,
  20 mg/12.5 mg, 20 mg/
  25 mg

LITHIUM
LITH ee um
TRADE NAME(S):
  Eskalith, Eskalith CR,
  Lithotabs, Lithobid
THERAPEUTIC CLASS:
  Antipsychotic
GENERAL USES:
  Psychotic disorders
DOSAGE FORMS:
  Capsules: 150 mg,
  300 mg, 600 mg; Tablets:
  300 mg; Sustained-
  release tablets: 300 mg;
  Controlled-release tablets:
  450 mg; Syrup: 8 mEq or
  300 mg/5 mL

LODOXAMIDE
loe DOKS a mide
TRADE NAME(S):
  Alomide
THERAPEUTIC CLASS:
  Ocular agent
GENERAL USES:
  Allergic conjunctivitis
DOSAGE FORMS:
  Ophthalmic solution: 0.1%

LOMEFLOXACIN
loe me FLOKS a sin
TRADE NAME(S):
  Maxaquin
THERAPEUTIC CLASS:
  Anti-infective
GENERAL USES:
  Bacterial infections

DOSAGE FORMS:
Tablets: 400 mg

**LOPINAVIR/
RITONAVIR**
loe PIN a veer/ri TOE na veer
TRADE NAME(S):
Kaletra
THERAPEUTIC CLASS:
Antiviral
GENERAL USES:
HIV infection
DOSAGE FORMS:
Solution: 80 mg/20 mg
per mL; Tablets: 200 mg/
500 mg

LORATADINE
lor AT a deen
TRADE NAME(S):
Claritin
THERAPEUTIC CLASS:
Antihistamine
GENERAL USES:
Allergic rhinitis/hives
DOSAGE FORMS:
Tablets: 10 mg; Syrup:
1 mg/mL (240 mL);
Rapidly disintegrating
tablets: 10 mg

**LORATADINE/
PSEUDOEPHEDRINE**
lor AT a deen/soo doe e
FED rin
TRADE NAME(S):
Claritin-D, Claritin-D

24 Hour
THERAPEUTIC CLASS:
Antihistamine/
decongestant
GENERAL USES:
Allergic rhinitis
DOSAGE FORMS:
Tablets: 5 mg/120 mg (D),
10 mg/240 mg (D-24)

LORAZEPAM
lor A ze pam
TRADE NAME(S):
Ativan
THERAPEUTIC CLASS:
Antianxiety agent
GENERAL USES:
Anxiety, sedation
DOSAGE FORMS:
Tablets: 0.5 mg, 1 mg,
2 mg; Concentrated
solution: 2 mg/mL;
Injection: 2 mg, 4 mg,
8 mg, 20 mg, 40 mg

LOSARTAN
loe SAR tan
TRADE NAME(S):
Cozaar
THERAPEUTIC CLASS:
Antihypertensive
GENERAL USES:
Hypertension, diabetic
nephropathy
DOSAGE FORMS:
Tablets: 25 mg, 50 mg,
100 mg

LOSARTAN/HCTZ
loe SAR tan/hye droe klor oh THYE a zide

TRADE NAME(S):
Hyzaar

THERAPEUTIC CLASS:
Antihypertensive/diuretic

GENERAL USES:
Hypertension

DOSAGE FORMS:
Tablets: 50 mg/12.5 mg, 100 mg/25 mg

LOTEPREDNOL
loe te PRED nol

TRADE NAME(S):
Lotemax, Alrex

THERAPEUTIC CLASS:
Ocular agent

GENERAL USES:
Ocular inflammation, allergies

DOSAGE FORMS:
Ophthalmic suspension: 0.2%, 0.5%

LOTEPREDNOL/ TOBRAMYCIN
loe te PRED nol/toe bra MYE sin

TRADE NAME(S):
Zylet

THERAPEUTIC CLASS:
Ocular agent

GENERAL USES:
Ocular inflammation/ infection

DOSAGE FORMS:
Ophthalmic solution: 0.5%/0.3%

LOVASTATIN
LOE va sta tin

TRADE NAME(S):
Mevacor, Altocor

THERAPEUTIC CLASS:
Antilipemic

GENERAL USES:
Hyperlipidemia, atherosclerosis

DOSAGE FORMS:
Tablets: 10 mg, 20 mg, 40 mg; Extended-release tablets: 10 mg, 20 mg, 40 mg, 60 mg

LOVASTATIN/NIACIN
LOE va sta tin/NYE a sin

TRADE NAME(S):
Advicor

THERAPEUTIC CLASS:
Antilipemic

GENERAL USES:
Hyperlipidemia

DOSAGE FORMS:
Caplets: 20 mg/1 g, 20 mg/750 mg, 20 mg/ 500 mg

LOXAPINE
LOKS a peen

TRADE NAME(S):
Loxitane, Loxitane C

THERAPEUTIC CLASS:
Antipsychotic

GENERAL USES:
  Psychotic disorders
DOSAGE FORMS:
  Capsules: 5 mg,
  10 mg, 25 mg, 50 mg;
  Concentrated solution:
  25 mg/mL; Injection:
  500 mg

LUBIPROSTONE
loo bi PROS tone
TRADE NAME(S):
  Amitiza
THERAPEUTIC CLASS:
  Laxative
GENERAL USES:
  Chronic idiopathic
  constipation
DOSAGE FORMS:
  Capsules: 24 mcg

MAGNESIUM SULFATE
mag NEE zhum
TRADE NAME(S):
  Magnesium Sulfate
THERAPEUTIC CLASS:
  Electrolyte
GENERAL USES:
  Anticonvulsant,
  replacement
DOSAGE FORMS:
  Injection:10%,12.5%,50%

MAPROTILINE
ma PROE ti leen
TRADE NAME(S):
  Ludiomil

THERAPEUTIC CLASS:
  Antidepressant
GENERAL USES:
  Depression
DOSAGE FORMS:
  Tablets: 25 mg, 50 mg,
  75 mg

MARAVIROC
mah RAV er rock
TRADE NAME(S):
  Selzentry
THERAPEUTIC CLASS:
  Antiviral
GENERAL USES:
  HIV infection
DOSAGE FORMS:
  Tablets: 150 mg, 300 mg

MECASERMIN RINFABATE (rDNA ORIGIN)
mek a SER min
TRADE NAME(S):
  iPlex
THERAPEUTIC CLASS:
  Hormone
GENERAL USES:
  Growth failure in children
DOSAGE FORMS:
  Injection: 36 mg

MECASERMIN (rDNA ORIGIN)
mek a SER min
TRADE NAME(S):
  Increlex

THERAPEUTIC CLASS:
Hormone

GENERAL USES:
Growth failure in children

DOSAGE FORMS:
Injection: 40 mg

MECLIZINE
MEK li zeen

TRADE NAME(S):
Antivert, Antrizine, Vergon

THERAPEUTIC CLASS:
Antiemetic/antivertigo agent

GENERAL USES:
Motion sickness

DOSAGE FORMS:
Tablets: 12.5 mg, 25 mg, 50 mg; Capsules: 25 mg, 30 mg; Chewable tablets: 25 mg

MEDROXY-PROGESTERONE ACETATE
me DROKS ee proe JES te rone

TRADE NAME(S):
Provera, Cycrin, Amen

THERAPEUTIC CLASS:
Hormone (progestin)

GENERAL USES:
Amenorrhea, uterine bleeding

DOSAGE FORMS:
Tablets: 2.5 mg, 5 mg, 10 mg

MEDROXY-PROGESTERONE ACETATE
me DROKS ee proe JES te rone

TRADE NAME(S):
Depo-Provera, Depo-SubQ Provera 104

THERAPEUTIC CLASS:
Hormone (progestin)

GENERAL USES:
Contraception

DOSAGE FORMS:
Injection: 150 mg, 104 mg

MEFENAMIC ACID
me fe NAM ik

TRADE NAME(S):
Ponstel

THERAPEUTIC CLASS:
Anti-inflammatory/ analgesic

GENERAL USES:
Menstrual cramping and pain

DOSAGE FORMS:
Capsules: 250 mg

MEFLOQUINE
ME floe kwin

TRADE NAME(S):
Lariam

THERAPEUTIC CLASS:
Antimalarial

GENERAL USES:
Malaria treatment and prevention

DOSAGE FORMS:
Tablets: 250 mg

MEGESTROL ACETATE
me JES trole

TRADE NAME(S):
Megace, Megace ES

THERAPEUTIC CLASS:
Hormone (progestin)

GENERAL USES:
Appetite enhancement, breast/endometrium cancers (palliative)

DOSAGE FORMS:
Tablets: 20 mg, 40 mg;
Suspension: 40 mg/mL;
Concentrate: 625 mg/
5 mL

MELOXICAM
mel OKS i kam

TRADE NAME(S):
Mobic

THERAPEUTIC CLASS:
Anti-inflammatory/
analgesic

GENERAL USES:
Osteoarthritis, rheumatoid arthritis

DOSAGE FORMS:
Tablets: 7.5 mg;
Suspension: 7.5 mg/5 mL

MEMANTINE
me MAN teen

TRADE NAME(S):
Namenda

THERAPEUTIC CLASS:
Alzheimer's agent

GENERAL USES:
Alzheimer's

DOSAGE FORMS:
Tablets: 5 mg, 10 mg;
Solution: 2 mg/mL

MEPERIDINE
me PER i deen

TRADE NAME(S):
Demerol

THERAPEUTIC CLASS:
Analgesic (narcotic)

GENERAL USES:
Pain

DOSAGE FORMS:
Tablets: 50 mg, 100 mg;
Syrup: 50 mg/5 mL;
Injection: 25 mg, 50 mg,
75 mg, 100 mg

MEQUINOL/TRETINOIN
ME kwi nole/TRET i noyn

TRADE NAME(S):
Solage

THERAPEUTIC CLASS:
Skin agent (topical)

GENERAL USES:
Aging solar skin spots

DOSAGE FORMS:
Solution: 2%/0.01%

MEROPENEM
mer oh PEN em

TRADE NAME(S):
Merrem IV

THERAPEUTIC CLASS:
Anti-infective

GENERAL USES:
Bacterial infections
DOSAGE FORMS:
Injection: 500 mg, 1 g

MESALAMINE
me SAL a meen
TRADE NAME(S):
Asacol, Lialda, Pentasa, Rowasa Rectal
THERAPEUTIC CLASS:
GI agent
GENERAL USES:
Inflammatory bowel disease
DOSAGE FORMS:
Delayed-release tablets: 400 mg, 1.2 g; Controlled-release capsules: 250 mg; Rectal enema: 4 g/60 mL; Suppository (rectal): 500 mg

MESORIDAZINE
mez oh RID a zeen
TRADE NAME(S):
Serentil
THERAPEUTIC CLASS:
Antipsychotic
GENERAL USES:
Psychotic disorders
DOSAGE FORMS:
Tablets: 10 mg, 25 mg, 50 mg, 100 mg; Concentrated solution: 25 mg/mL; Injection: 25 mg

MESTRANOL/ NORETHINDRONE
MES tra nole/nor eth IN drone
TRADE NAME(S):
Genora 1/50, Nelova 1/50M, Norethin 1/50M, Norinyl 1+50, Necon 1/50, Ortho-Novum 1/50
THERAPEUTIC CLASS:
Contraceptive (monophasic)
GENERAL USES:
Contraception
DOSAGE FORMS:
Tablets: 50 mcg/1 mg

METAPROTERENOL
met a proe TER e nol
TRADE NAME(S):
Alupent
THERAPEUTIC CLASS:
Bronchodilator
GENERAL USES:
Bronchospasm, asthma
DOSAGE FORMS:
Tablets: 10 mg, 20 mg; Syrup: 10 mg/5 mL; Aerosol: 5 mL, 10 mL; Inhalation solution: 0.4%, 0.6%, 5%

METAXALONE
me TAKS a lone
TRADE NAME(S):
Skelaxin
THERAPEUTIC CLASS:
Skeletal muscle relaxant

GENERAL USES:
Musculoskeletal
conditions
DOSAGE FORMS:
Tablets: 800 mg

METFORMIN
met FOR min
TRADE NAME(S):
Fortamet, Glucophage,
Glucophage XR, Glumetza
THERAPEUTIC CLASS:
Antidiabetic
GENERAL USES:
Diabetes (type 2)
DOSAGE FORMS:
Tablets: 500 mg, 850 mg,
1000 mg; Extended-
release tablets: 100 mg,
500 mg, 750 mg, 1000 mg

METFORMIN/ GLIPIZIDE
met FOR min/GLIP i zide
TRADE NAME(S):
Metaglip
THERAPEUTIC CLASS:
Antidiabetic
GENERAL USES:
Diabetes
DOSAGE FORMS:
Tablets: 250 mg/2.5 mg,
500 mg/2.5 mg, 500 mg/
5 mg

METFORMIN/ PIOGLITAZONE
met FOR min/pye oh GLI ta
zone

TRADE NAME(S):
Actoplus Met
THERAPEUTIC CLASS:
Antidiabetic
GENERAL USES:
Diabetes
DOSAGE FORMS:
Tablets: 500 mg/15 mg,
850 mg/15 mg

METHIMAZOLE
meth IM a zole
TRADE NAME(S):
Tapazole
THERAPEUTIC CLASS:
Antithyroid agent
GENERAL USES:
Hyperthyroidism
DOSAGE FORMS:
Tablets: 5 mg, 10 mg

METHOCARBAMOL
meth oh KAR ba mole
TRADE NAME(S):
Robaxin
THERAPEUTIC CLASS:
Skeletal muscle
relaxant
GENERAL USES:
Musculoskeletal
conditions
DOSAGE FORMS:
Tablets: 500 mg, 750 mg

METHOTREXATE
meth oh TREKS ate

TRADE NAME(S):
Rheumatrex, Trexall
THERAPEUTIC CLASS:
Antineoplastic,
antirheumatic
GENERAL USES:
Cancer, rheumatoid
arthritis
DOSAGE FORMS:
Tablets: 2.5 mg, 5 mg,
7.5 mg, 10 mg, 15 mg;
Injection: 20 mg, 50 mg,
250 mg, 1 g

**METHOXY
POLYETHYLENE GLYCOL
EPOETIN BETA**
meth OX ee pol ee ETH
i leen GLY kol e POE e tin
BAY ta
TRADE NAME(S):
Mircera
THERAPEUTIC CLASS:
Hematological agent
GENERAL USES:
Anemia
DOSAGE FORMS:
Injection: 50 mcg,
75 mcg, 100 mcg,
150 mcg, 200 mcg,
250 mcg, 300 mcg,
400 mcg, 600 mcg,
800 mcg, 1000 mcg

METHYLDOPA
meth il DOE pa
TRADE NAME(S):
Aldomet

THERAPEUTIC CLASS:
Antihypertensive
GENERAL USES:
Hypertension
DOSAGE FORMS:
Tablets: 125 mg, 250 mg,
500 mg; Suspension:
250 mg/5 mL; Injection:
250 mg (methyldopate)

METHYLDOPA/HCTZ
meth il DOE pa/hye droe klor
oh THYE a zide
TRADE NAME(S):
Aldoril
THERAPEUTIC CLASS:
Antihypertensive/
diuretic
GENERAL USES:
Hypertension
DOSAGE FORMS:
Tablets: 250 mg/15 mg,
250 mg/25 mg, 500 mg/
30 mg, 500 mg/50 mg

METHYLNALTREXONE
meth il nal TREKS one
TRADE NAME(S):
Relistor
THERAPEUTIC CLASS:
GI agent
GENERAL USES:
Opioid-induced
constipation
DOSAGE FORMS:
Injection: 12 mg

METHYLPHENIDATE
meth il FEN i date

TRADE NAME(S):
Concerta, Metadate, Metadate CD, Ritalin, Ritalin LA, Methylin

THERAPEUTIC CLASS:
CNS stimulant

GENERAL USES:
ADHD, narcolepsy

DOSAGE FORMS:
Tablets: 5 mg, 10 mg, 20 mg; Sustained-release tablets or capsules: 20 mg; Extended-release tablets: 10 mg, 18 mg, 20 mg, 27 mg, 36 mg, 54 mg; Extended-release capsules: 10 mg, 20 mg, 30 mg, 40 mg; Oral solution: 5 mg/5 mL, 10 mg/5 mL; Chewable tablets: 2.5 mg, 5 mg, 10 mg

METHYLPHENIDATE (TRANSDERMAL)
meth il FEN i date

TRADE NAME(S):
Daytrana

THERAPEUTIC CLASS:
CNS stimulant

GENERAL USES:
ADHD (age 6 to 12 yr)

DOSAGE FORMS:
Patch: 15 mg

METHYLPREDNISOLONE
meth il pred NIS oh lone

TRADE NAME(S):
Medrol

THERAPEUTIC CLASS:
Glucocorticoid

GENERAL USES:
Endocrine, skin, blood disorders

DOSAGE FORMS:
Tablets: 2 mg, 4 mg, 8 mg, 16 mg, 24 mg, 32 mg

METHYLPREDNISOLONE ACETATE
meth il pred NIS oh lone

TRADE NAME(S):
Depo-Medrol, Depoject, Depopred

THERAPEUTIC CLASS:
Glucocorticoid

GENERAL USES:
Endocrine, skin, blood disorders

DOSAGE FORMS:
Injection: 40 mg, 80 mg, 100 mg, 200 mg, 400 mg

METHYLPREDNISOLONE SODIUM SUCCINATE
meth il pred NIS oh lone

TRADE NAME(S):
A-Methapred, Solu-Medrol

THERAPEUTIC CLASS:
Glucocorticoid

GENERAL USES:
Endocrine, skin, blood disorders

DOSAGE FORMS:
Injection: 40 mg, 125 mg, 500 mg, 1 g, 2g

METHYSERGIDE
meth i SER jide

TRADE NAME(S):
Sansert

THERAPEUTIC CLASS:
Antimigraine agent

GENERAL USES:
Migraines

DOSAGE FORMS:
Tablets: 2 mg

METIPRANOLOL
met i PRAN oh lol

TRADE NAME(S):
OptiPranolol

THERAPEUTIC CLASS:
Ocular agent

GENERAL USES:
Glaucoma/ocular hypertension

DOSAGE FORMS:
Ophthalmic solution: 0.3%

METOCLOPRAMIDE
met oh KLOE pra mide

TRADE NAME(S):
Reglan, Clopra, Maxolon, Octamide, Reclomide

THERAPEUTIC CLASS:
Antiemetic

GENERAL USES:
Nausea, vomiting

DOSAGE FORMS:
Tablets: 5 mg, 10 mg;
Syrup: 5 mg/5 mL;
Concentrated solution:
10 mg/mL; Injection:
10 mg, 50 mg,
150 mg

METOLAZONE
me TOLE a zone

TRADE NAME(S):
Mykrox, Zaroxolyn

THERAPEUTIC CLASS:
Diuretic

GENERAL USES:
CHF-related edema, hypertension

DOSAGE FORMS:
Tablets: 0.5 mg, 2.5 mg, 5 mg, 10 mg

METOPROLOL
me toe PROE lole

TRADE NAME(S):
Lopressor, Toprol-XL

THERAPEUTIC CLASS:
Antihypertensive, antianginal, cardiac agent

GENERAL USES:
Hypertension, angina, MI

DOSAGE FORMS:
Tablets: 25 mg, 50 mg, 100 mg; Extended-release tablets: 25 mg, 50 mg, 100 mg, 200 mg; Injection: 5 mg

METOPROLOL/HCTZ
me toe PROE lole/hye dro
klor oh THYE a zide
TRADE NAME(S):
  Lopressor HCT
THERAPEUTIC CLASS:
  Antihypertensive/
  diuretic
GENERAL USES:
  Hypertension
DOSAGE FORMS:
  Tablets: 50 mg/25 mg,
  100 mg/25 mg, 100 mg/
  50 mg

METRONIDAZOLE
me troe NI da zole
TRADE NAME(S):
  Flagyl, Flagyl IV
THERAPEUTIC CLASS:
  Anti-infective
GENERAL USES:
  Bacterial infections,
  gastric ulcers
DOSAGE FORMS:
  Tablets: 250 mg, 500 mg;
  Extended-release tablets:
  750 mg; Capsules:
  375 mg; Injection: 500 mg

**METRONIDAZOLE
(TOPICAL)**
me troe NI da zole
TRADE NAME(S):
  MetroGel, MetroLotion,
  Noritate
THERAPEUTIC CLASS:
  Anti-infective (topical)

GENERAL USES:
  Rosacea acne
DOSAGE FORMS:
  Gel and Lotion: 0.75%;
  Cream: 1%

**METRONIDAZOLE
(VAGINAL)**
me troe NI da zole
TRADE NAME(S):
  MetroGel-Vaginal
THERAPEUTIC CLASS:
  Vaginal anti-infective
GENERAL USES:
  Bacterial vaginosis
DOSAGE FORMS:
  Gel: 0.75%

MEXILETINE
meks IL e teen
TRADE NAME(S):
  Mexitil
THERAPEUTIC CLASS:
  Antiarrhythmic
GENERAL USES:
  Arrhythmias,
  tachycardia
DOSAGE FORMS:
  Capsules: 150 mg,
  200 mg, 250 mg

MEZLOCILLIN
mez loe SIL in
TRADE NAME(S):
  Mezlin
THERAPEUTIC CLASS:
  Anti-infective

GENERAL USES:
Bacterial infections
DOSAGE FORMS:
Injection: 1 g, 2 g, 3 g,
4 g, 20 g

MICAFUNGIN SODIUM
mi ka FUN gin
TRADE NAME(S):
Mycamine
THERAPEUTIC CLASS:
Antifungal
GENERAL USES:
Candida infections
DOSAGE FORMS:
Injection: 50 mg

MICONAZOLE
mi KON a zole
TRADE NAME(S):
Monistat-3, Monistat-
Derm
THERAPEUTIC CLASS:
Vaginal antifungal
GENERAL USES:
Vaginal candidiasis
DOSAGE FORMS:
Vaginal suppository:
200 mg; Topical cream:
2%

MICONAZOLE/ZINC OXIDE/WHITE PETROLATUM
mi KON a zole
TRADE NAME(S):
Vusion

THERAPEUTIC CLASS:
Dermatological agent
GENERAL USES:
Diaper dermatitis/
candidiasis
DOSAGE FORMS:
Ointment: 30 g

MIDAZOLAM
mi DAZ oh lam
TRADE NAME(S):
Versed
THERAPEUTIC CLASS:
Sedative
GENERAL USES:
Preoperative sedation
DOSAGE FORMS:
Syrup: 2 mg/mL;
Injection: 2 mg, 5 mg,
10 mg, 25 mg, 50 mg

MIFEPRISTONE
mi FE pris tone
TRADE NAME(S):
Mifeprex
THERAPEUTIC CLASS:
Progesterone
antagonist
GENERAL USES:
Abortifacient
DOSAGE FORMS:
Tablets: 200 mg

MIGLITOL
MIG li tol
TRADE NAME(S):
Glyset

THERAPEUTIC CLASS:
  Antidiabetic
GENERAL USES:
  Diabetes (type 2)
DOSAGE FORMS:
  Tablets: 25 mg, 50 mg,
  100 mg

MIGLUSTAT
MIG loo stat
TRADE NAME(S):
  Zavesca
THERAPEUTIC CLASS:
  Enzyme inhibitor
GENERAL USES:
  Gaucher's disease
DOSAGE FORMS:
  Capsules: 100 mg

MINOCYCLINE
mi noe SYE kleen
TRADE NAME(S):
  Dynacin, Vectrin, Minocin,
  Solodyn
THERAPEUTIC CLASS:
  Anti-infective
GENERAL USES:
  Bacterial infections
DOSAGE FORMS:
  Tablets and Capsules:
  50 mg, 75 mg, 100 mg;
  Extended-release tablets:
  45 mg, 90 mg, 135 mg;
  Suspension: 50 mg/5 mL

MINOXIDIL
mi NOKS i dil

TRADE NAME(S):
  Loniten
THERAPEUTIC CLASS:
  Antihypertensive
GENERAL USES:
  Hypertension
DOSAGE FORMS:
  Tablets: 2.5 mg, 10 mg

MIRTAZAPINE
mir TAZ a peen
TRADE NAME(S):
  Remeron
THERAPEUTIC CLASS:
  Antidepressant
GENERAL USES:
  Depression
DOSAGE FORMS:
  Tablets and Orally
  disintegrating tablets:
  7.5 mg (orally
  disintegrating only),
  15 mg, 30 mg, 45 mg

MISOPROSTOL
mye soe PROST ole
TRADE NAME(S):
  Cytotec
THERAPEUTIC CLASS:
  Gastric protectant
GENERAL USES:
  Prevention of NSAID
  gastric ulcer
DOSAGE FORMS:
  Tablets: 100 mcg,
  200 mcg

MODAFANIL
moe DAF i nil
TRADE NAME(S):
Provigil
THERAPEUTIC CLASS:
CNS stimulant
GENERAL USES:
Narcolepsy, improve
fatigue associated with
sleep apnea and sleep
disorders
DOSAGE FORMS:
Tablets: 100 mg, 200 mg

MOEXIPRIL
mo EKS i pril
TRADE NAME(S):
Univasc
THERAPEUTIC CLASS:
Antihypertensive, cardiac
agent
GENERAL USES:
Hypertension, left
ventricular dysfunction
DOSAGE FORMS:
Tablets: 7.5 mg, 15 mg

MOEXIPRIL/HCTZ
mo EKS i pril/hye droe klor
oh THYE a zide
TRADE NAME(S):
Uniretic
THERAPEUTIC CLASS:
Antihypertensive/
diuretic
GENERAL USES:
Hypertension

DOSAGE FORMS:
Tablets: 15 mg/25 mg,
7.5 mg/12.5 mg

MOLINDONE
moe LIN done
TRADE NAME(S):
Moban
THERAPEUTIC CLASS:
Antipsychotic
GENERAL USES:
Psychotic disorders
DOSAGE FORMS:
Tablets: 5 mg, 10 mg,
25 mg, 50 mg

MOMETASONE (NASAL)
moe MET a sone
TRADE NAME(S):
Nasonex
THERAPEUTIC CLASS:
Corticosteroid (nasal)
GENERAL USES:
Allergies
DOSAGE FORMS:
Nasal spray: 50 mcg/
spray

MOMETASONE (TOPICAL)
moe MET a sone
TRADE NAME(S):
Elocon
THERAPEUTIC CLASS:
Corticosteroid (topical)
GENERAL USES:
Various skin
conditions

DOSAGE FORMS:
Ointment, Cream, and
Lotion: 0.1%

MOMETASONE FUROATE (ORAL INHALER)
moe MET a sone
FYOOR oh ate
TRADE NAME(S):
Asmanex
THERAPEUTIC CLASS:
Corticosteroid
GENERAL USES:
Asthma
DOSAGE FORMS:
Oral inhalation: 220 mcg/
inhalation

MONTELUKAST
mon te LOO kast
TRADE NAME(S):
Singulair
THERAPEUTIC CLASS:
Bronchodilator
GENERAL USES:
Asthma prevention and
treatment, seasonal
allergies
DOSAGE FORMS:
Tablets: 10 mg; Chewable
tablets: 4 mg, 5 mg;
Granules: 4 mg

MORICIZINE
mor I siz een
TRADE NAME(S):
Ethmozine

THERAPEUTIC CLASS:
Antiarrhythmic
GENERAL USES:
Arrhythmias
DOSAGE FORMS:
Tablets: 200 mg, 250 mg,
300 mg

MORPHINE
MOR feen
TRADE NAME(S):
Avinza, MS Contin,
Oramorph SR, Kadian,
Roxanol, Duramorph,
Infumorph
THERAPEUTIC CLASS:
Analgesic (narcotic)
GENERAL USES:
Pain
DOSAGE FORMS:
Tablets: 15 mg, 30 mg;
Controlled-release tablets:
15 mg, 30 mg, 60 mg,
100 mg, 200 mg; Soluble
tablets: 10 mg, 15 mg,
30 mg; Capsules: 15 mg,
30 mg; Sustained-release
capsules: 20 mg, 50 mg,
100 mg; Extended-release
capsules: 30 mg, 60 mg,
90 mg, 120 mg; Solution:
various concentrations;
Injection: various
concentrations

MORPHINE SULFATE (LIPOSOMAL)
MOR feen

TRADE NAME(S):
DepoDur

THERAPEUTIC CLASS:
Analgesic (narcotic)

GENERAL USES:
Major pain following
surgery (single-dose
administration)

DOSAGE FORMS:
Injection: 10 mg, 15 mg,
20 mg

MOXIFLOXACIN
moks i FLOKS a sin

TRADE NAME(S):
Avelox

THERAPEUTIC CLASS:
Anti-infective

GENERAL USES:
Bacterial infections

DOSAGE FORMS:
Tablets: 400 mg;
Injection: 400 mg

MOXIFLOXACIN
(OCULAR)
moks i FLOKS a sin

TRADE NAME(S):
Vigamox

THERAPEUTIC CLASS:
Ocular agent (anti-
infective)

GENERAL USES:
Bacterial
conjunctivitis

DOSAGE FORMS:
Ophthalmic solution:
0.5%

MUPIROCIN
myoo PEER oh sin

TRADE NAME(S):
Bactroban

THERAPEUTIC CLASS:
Anti-infective (topical)

GENERAL USES:
Impetigo, skin infections

DOSAGE FORMS:
Ointment and Cream: 2%

MYCOPHENOLATE
MOFETIL
mye koe FEN oh late MOE
feh till

TRADE NAME(S):
CellCept

THERAPEUTIC CLASS:
Immunosuppressant

GENERAL USES:
Prevent organ transplant
rejection

DOSAGE FORMS:
Capsules: 250 mg;
Tablets: 180 mg, 360 mg,
500 mg; Suspension:
200 mg/mL

NABILONE
NA bi lone

TRADE NAME(S):
Cesamet

THERAPEUTIC CLASS:
Antiemetic

GENERAL USES:
Chemotherapy-related
nausea and vomiting

DOSAGE FORMS:
  Capsules: 1 mg

NABUMETONE
na BYOO me tone
TRADE NAME(S):
  Relafen
THERAPEUTIC CLASS:
  Anti-inflammatory/
  analgesic
GENERAL USES:
  Osteoarthritis, rheumatoid
  arthritis
DOSAGE FORMS:
  Tablets: 500 mg, 750 mg

NADOLOL
nay DOE lole
TRADE NAME(S):
  Corgard
THERAPEUTIC CLASS:
  Antihypertensive,
  antianginal
GENERAL USES:
  Hypertension, angina
DOSAGE FORMS:
  Tablets: 20 mg, 40 mg,
  80 mg, 120 mg,
  160 mg

NAFCILLIN
naf SIL in
TRADE NAME(S):
  Unipen, Nallpen
THERAPEUTIC CLASS:
  Anti-infective
GENERAL USES:
  Bacterial infections

DOSAGE FORMS:
  Capsules: 250 mg;
  Injection: 500 mg, 1 g,
  2 g, 10 g

NAFTIFINE
NAF ti feen
TRADE NAME(S):
  Naftin
THERAPEUTIC CLASS:
  Antifungal (topical)
GENERAL USES:
  Athlete's foot, jock itch,
  ringworm
DOSAGE FORMS:
  Cream and Gel: 1%

NALOXONE
nal OKS one
TRADE NAME(S):
  Narcan
THERAPEUTIC CLASS:
  Antidote
GENERAL USES:
  Reversal of opioid effects
DOSAGE FORMS:
  Injection: 0.04 mg,
  0.4 mg, 0.8 mg, 2 mg,
  4 mg, 10 mg

NALTREXONE
nal TREKS one
TRADE NAME(S):
  Depade, ReVia, Vivitrol
THERAPEUTIC CLASS:
  Narcotic antagonist
GENERAL USES:
  Treatment of alcohol

dependence; blocks
narcotic effects
DOSAGE FORMS:
  Tablets: 25 mg, 50 mg,
  100 mg; Injection: 380 mg

NAPHAZOLINE
naf AZ oh leen
TRADE NAME(S):
  AK-Con, Albalon,
  Vasocon
THERAPEUTIC CLASS:
  Ocular agent
GENERAL USES:
  Ocular irritation
DOSAGE FORMS:
  Ophthalmic solution: 0.1%

NAPROXEN
na PROKS en
TRADE NAME(S):
  Anaprox DS, Aleve,
  Naprelan
THERAPEUTIC CLASS:
  Anti-inflammatory/
  analgesic
GENERAL USES:
  Osteoarthritis, rheumatoid
  arthritis, pain
DOSAGE FORMS:
  Tablets: 200 mg, 250 mg,
  375 mg, 500 mg;
  Delayed-release or
  Controlled-release
  tablets: 375 mg, 500 mg;
  Suspension: 125 mg/
  5 mL

NARATRIPTAN
NAR a trip tan
TRADE NAME(S):
  Amerge
THERAPEUTIC CLASS:
  Antimigraine agent
GENERAL USES:
  Migraines
DOSAGE FORMS:
  Tablets: 1 mg, 2.5 mg

NATALIZUMAB
nay tal IZ oo mab
TRADE NAME(S):
  Tysabri
THERAPEUTIC CLASS:
  Monoclonal antibody
GENERAL USES:
  Multiple sclerosis
DOSAGE FORMS:
  Injection: 300 mg

NATEGLINIDE
na te GLYE nide
TRADE NAME(S):
  Starlix
THERAPEUTIC CLASS:
  Antidiabetic
GENERAL USES:
  Diabetes (type 2)
DOSAGE FORMS:
  Tablets: 60 mg,
  120 mg

NEBIVOLOL
ne BIV oh lol
TRADE NAME(S):
  Bystolic

Therapeutic Class:
  Antihypertensive
General Uses:
  Hypertension
Dosage Forms:
  Tablets: 2.5 mg, 5 mg,
  10 mg

NEDOCROMIL
ne doe KROE mil
Trade Name(s):
  Tilade
Therapeutic Class:
  Respiratory inhalant
General Uses:
  Asthma
Dosage Forms:
  Inhaler: 1.75 mg/
  inhalation

NEFAZODONE
nef AY zoe done
Trade Name(s):
  Serzone
Therapeutic Class:
  Antidepressant
General Uses:
  Depression
Dosage Forms:
  Tablets: 50 mg, 100 mg,
  150 mg, 200 mg, 250 mg

NELARABINE
nel AY ra been
Trade Name(s):
  Arranon
Therapeutic Class:
  Antineoplastic

General Uses:
  Lymphoblastic lymphoma,
  leukemia
Dosage Forms:
  Injection: 250 mg

NELFINAVIR
nel FIN a veer
Trade Name(s):
  Viracept
Therapeutic Class:
  Antiviral
General Uses:
  HIV infection
Dosage Forms:
  Tablets: 250 mg, 625 mg;
  Powder: 50 mg/g

NEPAFENAC
ne pa FEN ak
Trade Name(s):
  Nevanac
Therapeutic Class:
  Ocular agent
General Uses:
  Pain and inflammation
  after cataract surgery
Dosage Forms:
  Ophthalmic suspension:
  0.1%

NESIRITIDE CITRATE
ni SIR i tide
Trade Name(s):
  Natrecor
Therapeutic Class:
  Cardiac agent

GENERAL USES:
CHF
DOSAGE FORMS:
Injection: 1.5 mg

NEVIRAPINE
ne VYE ra peen
TRADE NAME(S):
Viramune
THERAPEUTIC CLASS:
Antiviral
GENERAL USES:
HIV infection
DOSAGE FORMS:
Tablets: 200 mg;
Suspension:
50 mg/5 mL

NIACIN
(NICOTINIC ACID)
NYE a sin
TRADE NAME(S):
Niaspan
THERAPEUTIC CLASS:
Antilipemic
GENERAL USES:
Hyperlipidemia
DOSAGE FORMS:
Extended-release
tablets: 500 mg, 750 mg,
1000 mg

NICARDIPINE
nye KAR de peen
TRADE NAME(S):
Cardene, Cardene SR,
Cardene IV

THERAPEUTIC CLASS:
Antihypertensive,
antianginal
GENERAL USES:
Hypertension, angina
DOSAGE FORMS:
Capsules: 20 mg, 30 mg;
Sustained-release
capsules: 30 mg, 45 mg,
60 mg; Injection: 25 mg

NIFEDIPINE
nye FED i peen
TRADE NAME(S):
Adalat, Procardia, Adalat
CC, Procardia XL
THERAPEUTIC CLASS:
Antihypertensive
(sustained release),
antianginal
GENERAL USES:
Hypertension, angina
DOSAGE FORMS:
Capsules: 10 mg, 20 mg;
Extended-release tablets:
30 mg, 60 mg, 90 mg

NILOTINIB
nye LOE ti nib
TRADE NAME(S):
Tasigna
THERAPEUTIC CLASS:
Antineoplastic
GENERAL USES:
Leukemia
DOSAGE FORMS:
Capsules: 200 mg

NILUTAMIDE
ni LOO ta mide
TRADE NAME(S):
 Nilandron
THERAPEUTIC CLASS:
 Antiandrogen/
 antineoplastic
GENERAL USES:
 Prostate cancer
DOSAGE FORMS:
 Tablets: 50 mg

NIMODIPINE
nye MOE di peen
TRADE NAME(S):
 Nimotop
THERAPEUTIC CLASS:
 Cardiac agent
GENERAL USES:
 Brain hemorrhage
DOSAGE FORMS:
 Capsules: 30 mg

NISOLDIPINE
NYE sole di peen
TRADE NAME(S):
 Sular
THERAPEUTIC CLASS:
 Antihypertensive
GENERAL USES:
 Hypertension
DOSAGE FORMS:
 Extended-release
 tablets: 10 mg,
 20 mg, 30 mg,
 40 mg

NITAZOXANIDE
nye ta ZOKS a nide
TRADE NAME(S):
 Alinia
THERAPEUTIC CLASS:
 Anti-infective
GENERAL USES:
 Infectious diarrhea
DOSAGE FORMS:
 Suspension: 100 mg/
 5 mL

NITROFURANTOIN
nye troe fyoor AN toyn
TRADE NAME(S):
 Furadantin, Macrobid,
 Macrodantin
THERAPEUTIC CLASS:
 Anti-infective
GENERAL USES:
 Urinary tract infections
DOSAGE FORMS:
 Capsules: 25 mg, 50 mg,
 100 mg; Oral suspension:
 25 mg/5 mL

**NITROGLYCERIN
(INJECTION)**
nye troe GLI ser in
TRADE NAME(S):
 Tridil, Nitro-Bid IV
THERAPEUTIC CLASS:
 Antianginal
GENERAL USES:
 Angina
DOSAGE FORMS:
 Injection: 5 mg, 25 mg,
 50 mg, 100 mg

NITROGLYCERIN (SUBLINGUAL)

nye troe GLI ser in

TRADE NAME(S):
NitroQuick, Nitrostat, Nitrolingual, Nitrotab

THERAPEUTIC CLASS:
Antianginal

GENERAL USES:
Angina

DOSAGE FORMS:
Sublingual tablets: 0.3 mg, 0.4 mg, 0.6 mg; Spray: 0.4 mg/spray

NITROGLYCERIN (SUSTAINED RELEASE)

nye troe GLI ser in

TRADE NAME(S):
Nitrong, Nitroglyn, Nitro-Time

THERAPEUTIC CLASS:
Antianginal

GENERAL USES:
Angina

DOSAGE FORMS:
Sustained-release tablets: 2.6 mg, 6.5 mg, 9 mg; Sustained-release capsules: 2.5 mg, 6.5 mg, 9 mg, 13 mg

NITROGLYCERIN (TOPICAL)

nye troe GLI ser in

TRADE NAME(S):
Nitrol, Nitro-Bid

THERAPEUTIC CLASS:
Antianginal (topical)

GENERAL USES:
Angina

DOSAGE FORMS:
Ointment: 2%

NITROGLYCERIN (TRANSDERMAL)

nye troe GLI ser in

TRADE NAME(S):
Minitran, Nitro-Dur, Transderm-Nitro, Deponit

THERAPEUTIC CLASS:
Antianginal

GENERAL USES:
Angina

DOSAGE FORMS:
Release rate (mg/hr): 0.1 mg, 0.2 mg, 0.3 mg, 0.4 mg, 0.6 mg, 0.8 mg

NITROGLYCERIN (TRANSMUCOSAL-BUCCAL)

nye troe GLI ser in

TRADE NAME(S):
Nitrogard

THERAPEUTIC CLASS:
Antianginal

GENERAL USES:
Angina

DOSAGE FORMS:
Controlled-release tablets: 2 mg, 3 mg

NIZATIDINE
ni ZA ti deen

Trade Name(s):
Axid AR, Axid

Therapeutic Class:
Antiulcer agent

General Uses:
Duodenal ulcer, GERD,
heartburn (OTC)

Dosage Forms:
Tablets: 75 mg; Capsules:
150 mg, 300 mg

NORETHINDRONE
nor eth IN drone

Trade Name(s):
Micronor, Nor-QD

Therapeutic Class:
Contraceptive (progestin
only)

General Uses:
Contraception

Dosage Forms:
Tablets: 0.35 mg

NORETHINDRONE ACETATE
nor eth IN drone

Trade Name(s):
Aygestin

Therapeutic Class:
Hormone (progestin)

General Uses:
Amenorrhea,
endometriosis

Dosage Forms:
Tablets: 5 mg

NORFLOXACIN (OCULAR)
nor FLOKS a sin

Trade Name(s):
Chibroxin

Therapeutic Class:
Ocular agent (anti-
infective)

General Uses:
Ocular infections

Dosage Forms:
Ophthalmic solution:
3 mg/mL

NORFLOXACIN (ORAL)
nor FLOKS a sin

Trade Name(s):
Noroxin

Therapeutic Class:
Anti-infective

General Uses:
Bacterial infections

Dosage Forms:
Tablets: 400 mg

NORGESTREL
nor JES trel

Trade Name(s):
Ovrette

Therapeutic Class:
Contraceptive (progestin
only)

General Uses:
Contraception

Dosage Forms:
Tablets: 0.075 mg

NORTRIPTYLINE
nor TRIP ti leen

TRADE NAME(S):
Aventyl, Pamelor

THERAPEUTIC CLASS:
Antidepressant

GENERAL USES:
Depression

DOSAGE FORMS:
Capsules: 10 mg,
25 mg, 50 mg,
75 mg; Solution:
10 mg/5 mL

NYSTATIN (ORAL)
nye STAT in

TRADE NAME(S):
Nilstat, Mycostatin

THERAPEUTIC CLASS:
Antifungal

GENERAL USES:
Oral fungal infections
(candidiasis)

DOSAGE FORMS:
Suspension:
100,000 units/mL;
Troches: 200,000 units;
Tablets: 500,000 units

NYSTATIN (VAGINAL)
nye STAT in

TRADE NAME(S):
Nystatin

THERAPEUTIC CLASS:
Vaginal antifungal

GENERAL USES:
Vaginal candidiasis

DOSAGE FORMS:
Vaginal tablets:
100,000 units

OCTREOTIDE
ok TREE oh tide

TRADE NAME(S):
Sandostatin, Sandostatin
LAR Depot

THERAPEUTIC CLASS:
Hormone

GENERAL USES:
Acromegaly, carcinoid
tumors

DOSAGE FORMS:
Injection: 0.05 mg,
0.1 mg, 0.5 mg, 1 mg,
5 mg, 10 mg, 20 mg,
30 mg

OFLOXACIN
oh FLOKS a sin

TRADE NAME(S):
Floxin

THERAPEUTIC CLASS:
Anti-infective

GENERAL USES:
Bacterial infections

DOSAGE FORMS:
Tablets: 200 mg, 300 mg,
400 mg; Injection:
200 mg, 400 mg

OFLOXACIN (OCULAR)
oh FLOKS a sin

TRADE NAME(S):
Ocuflox

THERAPEUTIC CLASS:
Ocular agent (anti-infective)

GENERAL USES:
Ocular infections

DOSAGE FORMS:
Ophthalmic solution: 3 mg/mL

OFLOXACIN (OTIC)
oh FLOKS a sin

TRADE NAME(S):
Floxin Otic

THERAPEUTIC CLASS:
Anti-infective (Otic)

GENERAL USES:
Otitis externa

DOSAGE FORMS:
Otic solution: 0.3%

OLANZAPINE
oh LAN za peen

TRADE NAME(S):
Zyprexa

THERAPEUTIC CLASS:
Antipsychotic

GENERAL USES:
Psychotic disorders

DOSAGE FORMS:
Tablets: 2.5 mg, 5 mg, 7.5 mg, 10 mg, 15 mg, 20 mg; Orally disintegrating tablets: 5 mg, 10 mg, 15 mg, 20 mg; Injection: 10 mg

OLANZAPINE/ FLUOXETINE
oh LAN za peen/floo OKS e teen

TRADE NAME(S):
Symbyax

THERAPEUTIC CLASS:
Antipsychotic/ antidepressant

GENERAL USES:
Bipolar disorder/ depression

DOSAGE FORMS:
Capsules: 6 mg/25 mg, 6 mg/50 mg, 12 mg/ 25 mg, 12 mg/50 mg

OLMESARTAN
ole me SAR tan

TRADE NAME(S):
Benicar

THERAPEUTIC CLASS:
Antihypertensive

GENERAL USES:
Hypertension

DOSAGE FORMS:
Tablets: 5 mg, 20 mg, 40 mg

OLMESARTAN/HCTZ
ole me SAR tan/hye droe klor oh THYE a zide

TRADE NAME(S):
Benicar HCT

THERAPEUTIC CLASS:
Antihypertensive/ diuretic

GENERAL USES:
Hypertension
DOSAGE FORMS:
Tablets: 20 mg/12.5 mg,
40 mg/12.5 mg, 40 mg/
25 mg

OLOPATADINE (NASAL)
oh la PAT a deen
TRADE NAME(S):
Patanase
THERAPEUTIC CLASS:
Nasal agent
GENERAL USES:
Seasonal allergies
DOSAGE FORMS:
Nasal spray: 665 mcg/
spray

**OLOPATADINE
(OCULAR)**
oh la PAT a deen
TRADE NAME(S):
Patanol
THERAPEUTIC CLASS:
Ocular agent
GENERAL USES:
Allergic conjunctivitis
DOSAGE FORMS:
Ophthalmic solution: 0.1%

OLSALAZINE
ol SAL a zeen
TRADE NAME(S):
Dipentum
THERAPEUTIC CLASS:
GI agent

GENERAL USES:
Ulcerative colitis
DOSAGE FORMS:
Capsules: 250 mg

OMALIZUMAB
oh mah lye ZOO mab
TRADE NAME(S):
Xolair
THERAPEUTIC CLASS:
Antiasthma
GENERAL USES:
Asthma
DOSAGE FORMS:
Injection: 150 mg

**OMEGA-3 ACID ETHYL
ESTERS**
oh MEG a three AS id ETH il
ES ters
TRADE NAME(S):
Lovaza
THERAPEUTIC CLASS:
Fish oil
GENERAL USES:
Hypertriglyceridemia
DOSAGE FORMS:
Capsules: 1 g

OMEPRAZOLE
oh MEP ra zole
TRADE NAME(S):
Prilosec
THERAPEUTIC CLASS:
Gastric acid secretion
inhibitor
GENERAL USES:
Duodenal ulcer, GERD

Dosage Forms:
Delayed-release capsules:
10 mg, 20 mg, 40 mg;
Oral suspension: 20 mg

OMEPRAZOLE/SODIUM BICARBONATE
oh MEP ra zole/SOE dee um
bye KAR bo nate
Trade Name(s):
Zegerid
Therapeutic Class:
Gastric acid secretion
inhibitor/anti-ulcer agent
General Uses:
Duodenal ulcer, gastric
ulcer, GERD, erosive
esophagitis
Dosage Forms:
Capsules: 20 mg/
1100 mg, 40 mg/1100 mg;
Oral suspension (powder):
20 mg/1680 mg, 40 mg/
1680 mg

ONDANSETRON
on DAN se tron
Trade Name(s):
Zofran
Therapeutic Class:
Antiemetic
General Uses:
Surgical or chemotherapy
nausea/vomiting
Dosage Forms:
Tablets: 4 mg, 8 mg,
24 mg; Solution: 4 mg/

5 mL; Orally disintegrating
tablets: 4 mg, 8 mg;
Injection: 4 mg, 32 mg,
80 mg

ORLISTAT
OR li stat
Trade Name(s):
Xenical
Therapeutic Class:
Antiobesity
General Uses:
Obesity
Dosage Forms:
Capsules: 120 mg

ORPHENADRINE
or FEN a dreen
Trade Name(s):
Norflex
Therapeutic Class:
Skeletal muscle relaxant
General Uses:
Musculoskeletal
conditions
Dosage Forms:
Tablets and Sustained-
release tablets: 100 mg

OSELTAMIVIR
oh sel TAM i vir
Trade Name(s):
Tamiflu
Therapeutic Class:
Anti-influenza
General Uses:
Influenza A or B

DOSAGE FORMS:
Capsules: 30 mg, 45 mg, 75 mg; Oral suspension: 12 mg/mL

OXACILLIN
oks a SIL in
TRADE NAME(S):
Oxacillin
THERAPEUTIC CLASS:
Anti-infective
GENERAL USES:
Bacterial infections
DOSAGE FORMS:
Capsules: 250 mg, 500 mg; Solution: 250 mg/5 mL; Injection: 250 mg, 500 mg, 1 g, 2 g, 4 g, 10 g

OXALIPLATIN
oks AL i pla tin
TRADE NAME(S):
Eloxatin
THERAPEUTIC CLASS:
Antineoplastic
GENERAL USES:
Colon or rectal cancer (metastatic)
DOSAGE FORMS:
Injection: 50 mg, 100 mg

OXAPROZIN
oks a PROE zin
TRADE NAME(S):
Daypro

THERAPEUTIC CLASS:
Anti-inflammatory/ analgesic
GENERAL USES:
Osteoarthritis, rheumatoid arthritis
DOSAGE FORMS:
Tablets: 600 mg

OXAZEPAM
oks A ze pam
TRADE NAME(S):
Serax
THERAPEUTIC CLASS:
Antianxiety agent
GENERAL USES:
Anxiety
DOSAGE FORMS:
Tablets: 15 mg; Capsules: 10 mg, 15 mg, 30 mg

OXCARBAZEPINE
oks car BAZ e peen
TRADE NAME(S):
Trileptal
THERAPEUTIC CLASS:
Anticonvulsant
GENERAL USES:
Partial seizures (children)
DOSAGE FORMS:
Tablets: 150 mg, 300 mg, 600 mg; Suspension: 300 mg/5 mL

OXYBATE, SODIUM
OKS i bate
TRADE NAME(S):
Xyrem

THERAPEUTIC CLASS:
CNS depressant

GENERAL USES:
Cataplexy in narcolepsy

DOSAGE FORMS:
Solution: 500 mg/mL

OXYBUTYNIN
oks i BYOO ti nin

TRADE NAME(S):
Ditropan, Ditropan XL

THERAPEUTIC CLASS:
Antispasmodic

GENERAL USES:
Bladder instability

DOSAGE FORMS:
Tablets: 5 mg; Extended-release tablets: 5 mg, 10 mg, 15 mg; Syrup: 5 mg/5 mL

OXYBUTYNIN (TRANSDERMAL)
oks i BYOO ti nin

TRADE NAME(S):
Oxytrol

THERAPEUTIC CLASS:
Antispasmodic

GENERAL USES:
Bladder instability

DOSAGE FORMS:
Patch: 3.9 mg

OXYCODONE
oks i KOE done

TRADE NAME(S):
Percolone, Roxicodone, OxyContin, OxyIR, OxyFast

THERAPEUTIC CLASS:
Analgesic (narcotic)

GENERAL USES:
Pain

DOSAGE FORMS:
Tablets: 5 mg; Capsules: 5 mg; Controlled-release tablets: 10 mg, 20 mg, 40 mg, 80 mg; Solution: 5 mg/5 mL; Concentrated solution: 20 mg/mL

OXYCODONE/ ACETAMINOPHEN
oks ee KOE done/a seet a MIN oh fen

TRADE NAME(S):
Endocet, Percocet, Roxicet, Roxicet 5/500, Roxilox, Tylox

THERAPEUTIC CLASS:
Narcotic analgesic/ analgesic

GENERAL USES:
Pain

DOSAGE FORMS:
Tablets: 2.5 mg/325 mg, 5 mg/325 mg, 7.5 mg/ 325 mg, 7.5 mg/500 mg, 10 mg/325 mg, 10 mg/650 mg; Caplets: 5 mg/500 mg; Capsules: 5 mg/500 mg; Oral solution: 5 mg/325 mg per 5 mL

OXYMORPHONE
oks ee MOR fone
TRADE NAME(S):
Opana, Opana ER
THERAPEUTIC CLASS:
Narcotic analgesic
GENERAL USES:
Pain
DOSAGE FORMS:
Tablets: 5 mg, 10 mg;
Extended-release tablets:
5 mg, 7.5 mg, 10 mg,
15 mg, 20 mg, 30 mg,
40 mg; Injection: 1 mg

OXYTOCIN
oks i TOE sin
TRADE NAME(S):
Pitocin, Syntocinon
THERAPEUTIC CLASS:
Oxytocic
GENERAL USES:
Stimulant for labor
DOSAGE FORMS:
Injection: 5 units, 10 units,
100 units

PACLITAXEL
PAK li taks el
TRADE NAME(S):
Taxol
THERAPEUTIC CLASS:
Antineoplastic
GENERAL USES:
Various cancers
DOSAGE FORMS:
Injection: 30 mg,
100.2 mg, 150 mg,
300 mg

PACLITAXEL
(PROTEIN BOUND)
PAK li taks el
TRADE NAME(S):
Abraxane
THERAPEUTIC CLASS:
Antineoplastic
GENERAL USES:
Breast cancer
DOSAGE FORMS:
Injection: 100 mg

PALIFERMIN
pal ee FER min
TRADE NAME(S):
Kepivance
THERAPEUTIC CLASS:
Keratinocyte growth factor
GENERAL USES:
Mucositis
DOSAGE FORMS:
Injection: 6.25 mg

PALIPERIDONE
pal ee PER i done
TRADE NAME(S):
Invega
THERAPEUTIC CLASS:
Atypical antipsychotic
GENERAL USES:
Schizophrenia
DOSAGE FORMS:
Extended-release tablets:
3 mg, 6 mg, 9 mg

PALONOSETRON
pal oh NOE se tron
TRADE NAME(S):
Aloxi
THERAPEUTIC CLASS:
Antiemetic
GENERAL USES:
Chemotherapy-
induced nausea/
vomiting
DOSAGE FORMS:
Injection: 0.25 mg

PANCURONIUM
pan kyoo ROE nee um
TRADE NAME(S):
Pavulon
THERAPEUTIC CLASS:
Muscle relaxant
GENERAL USES:
Muscle relaxation for
intubation
DOSAGE FORMS:
Injection: 4 mg, 10 mg

PANITUMUMAB
pan ee TOO moo mab
TRADE NAME(S):
Vectibix
THERAPEUTIC CLASS:
Antineoplastic
GENERAL USES:
Colon cancer
DOSAGE FORMS:
Injection: 100 mg,
200 mg, 400 mg

PANTOPRAZOLE
pan TOE pra zole
TRADE NAME(S):
Protonix
THERAPEUTIC CLASS:
Gastric acid secretion
inhibitor
GENERAL USES:
Erosive esophagitis, GERD
DOSAGE FORMS:
Delayed-release tablets:
20 mg, 40 mg; Injection:
40 mg; Delayed-release
granules: 40 mg

PAPAVERINE
pa PAV er een
TRADE NAME(S):
Pavabid, Pavacot
THERAPEUTIC CLASS:
Cardiac agent
GENERAL USES:
Peripheral and cerebral
ischemia
DOSAGE FORMS:
Sustained-release
capsules: 150 mg

PARICALCITOL
pah ri KAL si tole
TRADE NAME(S):
Zemplar
THERAPEUTIC CLASS:
Vitamin D analog
GENERAL USES:
Secondary
hyperparathyroidism in

kidney disease
(children)
DOSAGE FORMS:
Injection: 5 mcg/mL;
Capsules: 1 mcg, 2 mcg,
4 mcg

PAROMOMYCIN
par oh moe MYE sin
TRADE NAME(S):
Humatin
THERAPEUTIC CLASS:
Antituberculosis
agent
GENERAL USES:
Tuberculosis
DOSAGE FORMS:
Capsules: 250 mg

PAROXETINE
pa ROKS e teen
TRADE NAME(S):
Paxil, Paxil CR,
Asimia
THERAPEUTIC CLASS:
Antidepressant
GENERAL USES:
Depression, OCD, panic,
social anxiety, PMDD,
PTSD
DOSAGE FORMS:
Tablets: 10 mg,
20 mg, 30 mg, 40 mg;
Controlled-release tablets:
12.5 mg, 25 mg, 37.5 mg;
Suspension: 10 mg/5 mL

PEGAPTANIB SODIUM
peg AP ta nib
TRADE NAME(S):
Macugen
THERAPEUTIC CLASS:
Ocular agent
GENERAL USES:
Macular degeneration
DOSAGE FORMS:
Injection: 0.3 mg

PEGINTERFERON ALFA-2a
peg in ter FEER on
TRADE NAME(S):
Pegasys
THERAPEUTIC CLASS:
Antiviral
GENERAL USES:
Hepatitis C
DOSAGE FORMS:
Injection: 180 mcg

PEGINTERFERON ALFA-2b
peg in ter FEER on
TRADE NAME(S):
Peg-Intron
THERAPEUTIC CLASS:
Antiviral
GENERAL USES:
Hepatitis C
DOSAGE FORMS:
Injection: 50 mcg,
80 mcg, 120 mcg,
150 mcg

PEGVISOMANT
peg VYE soe mant
TRADE NAME(S):
Somavert
THERAPEUTIC CLASS:
Growth hormone
antagonist
GENERAL USES:
Acromegaly
DOSAGE FORMS:
Injection: 10 mg, 15 mg,
20 mg

PEMETREXED
pem e TREKS ed
TRADE NAME(S):
Alimta
THERAPEUTIC CLASS:
Antineoplastic
GENERAL USES:
Various lung cancers
DOSAGE FORMS:
Injection: 500 mg

PENBUTOLOL
pen BYOO toe lole
TRADE NAME(S):
Levatol
THERAPEUTIC CLASS:
Antihypertensive
GENERAL USES:
Hypertension
DOSAGE FORMS:
Tablets: 20 mg

PENCICLOVIR
pen SYE kloe veer

TRADE NAME(S):
Denavir
THERAPEUTIC CLASS:
Antiviral (topical)
GENERAL USES:
Cold sores, oral
herpes
DOSAGE FORMS:
Cream: 1%

**PENICILLIN G
(AQUEOUS)**
pen i SIL in
TRADE NAME(S):
Penicillin G Potassium,
Pfizerpen
THERAPEUTIC CLASS:
Anti-infective
GENERAL USES:
Bacterial infections
DOSAGE FORMS:
Injection: 1 million units,
2 million units, 3 million
units, 5 million units,
10 million units, 20 million
units

**PENICILLIN G
BENZATHINE**
pen i SIL in jee BENZ a theen
TRADE NAME(S):
Bicillin LA, Permapen
THERAPEUTIC CLASS:
Anti-infective
GENERAL USES:
Bacterial infections
DOSAGE FORMS:
Injection: 600,000 units,

1.2 million units,
2.4 million units,
3 million units

PENICILLIN G PROCAINE
pen i SIL in jee PROE kane
TRADE NAME(S):
Wycillin
THERAPEUTIC CLASS:
Anti-infective
GENERAL USES:
Bacterial infections
DOSAGE FORMS:
Injection: 600,000 units,
1.2 million units,
2.4 million units

PENICILLIN VK
pen i SIL in
TRADE NAME(S):
Beepen-VK,
Pen-Vee K, Veetids
THERAPEUTIC CLASS:
Anti-infective
GENERAL USES:
Bacterial infections
DOSAGE FORMS:
Tablets: 250 mg, 500 mg;
Solution: 125 mg/5 mL,
250 mg/5 mL

**PENTAMIDINE
ISETHIONATE**
pen TAM i deen ice e THYE
ah nate
TRADE NAME(S):
Pentam 300, NebuPent

THERAPEUTIC CLASS:
Anti-infective
GENERAL USES:
Treatment or prevention
of pneumonia in HIV
infection
DOSAGE FORMS:
Injection and Aerosol:
300 mg

**PENTETATE CALCIUM
TRISODIUM**
PEN te tate
TRADE NAME(S):
Ca-DTPA
THERAPEUTIC CLASS:
Antidote
GENERAL USES:
Internal contamination
with plutonium,
americium, curium
DOSAGE FORMS:
Injection or Inhalation:
1000 mg

**PENTETATE ZINC
TRISODIUM**
PEN te tate
TRADE NAME(S):
Zn-DTPA
THERAPEUTIC CLASS:
Antidote
GENERAL USES:
Internal contamination
with plutonium,
americium, curium
DOSAGE FORMS:
Injection: 1000 mg

PENTOBARBITAL
pen toe BAR bi tal
TRADE NAME(S):
Nembutal
THERAPEUTIC CLASS:
Sedative/hypnotic
GENERAL USES:
Insomnia (short term therapy), pre-op sedative
DOSAGE FORMS:
Capsules: 50 mg, 100 mg; Elixir: 18.2 mg/5 mL; Injection: 1 g, 2.5 g

PENTOXIFYLLINE
pen toks I fi leen
TRADE NAME(S):
Pentoxil, Trental
THERAPEUTIC CLASS:
Blood viscosity reducer agent
GENERAL USES:
Intermittent claudication
DOSAGE FORMS:
Tablets, Controlled-release tablets, Extended-release tablets: 400 mg

PERMETHRIN
per METH rin
TRADE NAME(S):
Elimite, Acticin, Nix
THERAPEUTIC CLASS:
Scabicide/pediculicide (topical)
GENERAL USES:
Scabies, head lice

DOSAGE FORMS:
Cream: 5%; Lotion: 1%

PERPHENAZINE
per FEN a zeen
TRADE NAME(S):
Trilafon
THERAPEUTIC CLASS:
Antipsychotic
GENERAL USES:
Psychotic disorders
DOSAGE FORMS:
Tablets: 2 mg, 4 mg, 8 mg, 16 mg; Concentrated solution: 16 mg/5 mL; Injection: 5 mg

PERPHENAZINE/ AMITRIPTYLINE
per FEN a zeen/a mee TRIP ti leen
TRADE NAME(S):
Etrafon, Triavil
THERAPEUTIC CLASS:
Sedative/antidepressant
GENERAL USES:
Depression/anxiety
DOSAGE FORMS:
Tablets: 2 mg/10 mg, 2 mg/25 mg, 4 mg/ 25 mg, 4 mg/50 mg

PHENELZINE
FEN el zeen
TRADE NAME(S):
Nardil
THERAPEUTIC CLASS:
Antidepressant

GENERAL USES:
Depression
DOSAGE FORMS:
Tablets: 15 mg

PHENOBARBITAL
fee noe BAR bi tal
TRADE NAME(S):
Barbita, Solfoton
THERAPEUTIC CLASS:
Sedative/hypnotic,
anticonvulsant
GENERAL USES:
Seizures, insomnia (short
term therapy)
DOSAGE FORMS:
Tablets: 8 mg, 15 mg,
16 mg, 30 mg, 60 mg,
90 mg, 100 mg; Capsules:
16 mg; Elixir: 15 mg/
5 mL, 20 mg/5 mL;
Injection: 60 mg, 65 mg,
130 mg

PHENTERMINE
FEN ter meen
TRADE NAME(S):
Fastin, Zantryl, Adipex-P,
Ionamin
THERAPEUTIC CLASS:
Anorexiant
GENERAL USES:
Obesity
DOSAGE FORMS:
Tablets: 8 mg, 37.5 mg;
Capsules: 15 mg,
18.75 mg, 30 mg, 37.5 mg

PHENYTOIN
FEN i toyn
TRADE NAME(S):
Dilantin
THERAPEUTIC CLASS:
Anticonvulsant
GENERAL USES:
Seizures
DOSAGE FORMS:
Chewable tablets: 50 mg;
Suspension: 125 mg/
5 mL; Extended-release
tablets: 30 mg, 100 mg;
Prompt capsules: 100 mg;
Injection: 100 mg, 250 mg

PILOCARPINE (OCULAR)
pye loe KAR peen
TRADE NAME(S):
Isopto Carpine, Pilocar,
Akarpine, Pilostat
THERAPEUTIC CLASS:
Ocular agent
GENERAL USES:
Glaucoma
DOSAGE FORMS:
Ophthalmic solution:
0.25%, 0.5%, 1%, 2%,
3%, 4%, 5%, 6%, 8%,
10%; Ophthalmic gel: 4%

PILOCARPINE (ORAL)
pye loe KAR peen
TRADE NAME(S):
Salagen
THERAPEUTIC CLASS:
Saliva stimulant

GENERAL USES:
Saliva deficiency
DOSAGE FORMS:
Tablets: 5 mg

PIMECROLIMUS
pim e KROE li mus
TRADE NAME(S):
Elidel
THERAPEUTIC CLASS:
Anti-inflammatory agent
GENERAL USES:
Eczema
DOSAGE FORMS:
Cream: 1%

PIMOZIDE
PI moe zide
TRADE NAME(S):
Orap
THERAPEUTIC CLASS:
Antipsychotic
GENERAL USES:
Tourette's
DOSAGE FORMS:
Tablets: 2 mg

PINDOLOL
PIN doe lole
TRADE NAME(S):
Visken
THERAPEUTIC CLASS:
Antihypertensive
GENERAL USES:
Hypertension
DOSAGE FORMS:
Tablets: 5 mg, 10 mg

PIOGLITAZONE
pye oh GLI ta zone
TRADE NAME(S):
Actos
THERAPEUTIC CLASS:
Antidiabetic
GENERAL USES:
Diabetes (type 2)
DOSAGE FORMS:
Tablets: 15 mg, 30 mg,
45 mg

**PIOGLITAZONE/
GLIMEPIRIDE**
pye oh GLI ta zone/glye MEP
i ride
TRADE NAME(S):
Duetact
THERAPEUTIC CLASS:
Antidiabetic
GENERAL USES:
Diabetes (type 2)
DOSAGE FORMS:
Tablets: 30 mg/2 mg,
30 mg/4 mg

PIPERACILLIN
pi PER a sil in
TRADE NAME(S):
Pipracil
THERAPEUTIC CLASS:
Anti-infective
GENERAL USES:
Bacterial infections
DOSAGE FORMS:
Injection: 2 g, 3 g, 4 g,
40 g

PIPERACILLIN/ TAZOBACTAM

pi PER a sil in/ta zoe BAK tam

TRADE NAME(S):
Zosyn

THERAPEUTIC CLASS:
Anti-infective

GENERAL USES:
Bacterial infections

DOSAGE FORMS:
Injection: 2 g/0.25 g, 3 g/0.375 g, 4 g/0.5 g, 36 g/4.5 g

PIRBUTEROL

peer BYOO ter ole

TRADE NAME(S):
Maxair

THERAPEUTIC CLASS:
Bronchodilator

GENERAL USES:
Bronchospasm, asthma

DOSAGE FORMS:
Inhaler: 0.2 mg/inhalation

PIROXICAM

peer OKS i kam

TRADE NAME(S):
Feldene

THERAPEUTIC CLASS:
Anti-inflammatory/ analgesic

GENERAL USES:
Osteoarthritis, rheumatoid arthritis

DOSAGE FORMS:
Capsules: 10 mg, 20 mg

POLYETHYLENE GLYCOL

pol ee ETH i leen GLY kol

TRADE NAME(S):
MiraLax, GlycoLax

THERAPEUTIC CLASS:
Laxative

GENERAL USES:
Bowel cleansing

DOSAGE FORMS:
Powder for oral solution: 255 g, 527 g

POSACONAZOLE

poe sa KON a zole

TRADE NAME(S):
Noxafil

THERAPEUTIC CLASS:
Antifungal

GENERAL USES:
Fungal infections

DOSAGE FORMS:
Oral suspension: 40 mg/ mL

POTASSIUM CHLORIDE

poe TASS ee um KLOR ide

TRADE NAME(S):
K-Dur, Kaon-Cl, Klor-Con, Klotrix, Klorvess, K-Lyte, Micro-K

THERAPEUTIC CLASS:
Electrolyte (potassium)

GENERAL USES:
Potassium replacement

DOSAGE FORMS:
Controlled-release or Extended-release

tablets: 6.7 mEq, 8 mEq, 10 mEq; Effervescent tablets: 20 mEq, 25 mEq, 50 mEq; Liquid: 20 mEq, 30 mEq or 40 mEq/15 mL; Powder: 20 mEq, 25 mEq; Injection: various concentrations

PRAMIPEXOLE
pra mi PEKS ole
TRADE NAME(S):
Mirapex
THERAPEUTIC CLASS:
Antiparkinson agent
GENERAL USES:
Parkinson's disease
DOSAGE FORMS:
Tablets: 0.125 mg, 0.25 mg, 0.5 mg, 1 mg, 1.5 mg

PRAMLINTIDE ACETATE
PRAM lin tide
TRADE NAME(S):
Symlin
THERAPEUTIC CLASS:
Antidiabetic
GENERAL USES:
Diabetes
DOSAGE FORMS:
Injection: 3 mg

PRAVASTATIN
PRA va stat in
TRADE NAME(S):
Pravachol

THERAPEUTIC CLASS:
Antilipemic
GENERAL USES:
Hyperlipidemia
DOSAGE FORMS:
Tablets: 10 mg, 20 mg, 40 mg, 80 mg

PRAZOSIN
PRA zoe sin
TRADE NAME(S):
Minipress
THERAPEUTIC CLASS:
Antihypertensive
GENERAL USES:
Hypertension
DOSAGE FORMS:
Capsules: 1 mg, 2 mg, 5 mg

PRAZOSIN/ POLYTHIAZIDE
PRA zoe sin/pol i THYE a zide
TRADE NAME(S):
Minizide
THERAPEUTIC CLASS:
Antihypertensive/diuretic
GENERAL USES:
Hypertension
DOSAGE FORMS:
Capsules: 1 mg/0.5 mg, 2 mg/0.5 mg, 5 mg/ 0.5 mg

PREDNISOLONE (OCULAR)
pred NIS oh lone

TRADE NAME(S):
Pred Mild, Econopred,
Pred Forte

THERAPEUTIC CLASS:
Ocular agent (steroid)

GENERAL USES:
Ocular inflammation

DOSAGE FORMS:
Ophthalmic suspension
and Solution: 0.1%, 0.125%

PREDNISOLONE (ORAL)
pred NIS oh lone

TRADE NAME(S):
Orapred ODT, Prelone,
Delta-Cortef, Flo-Pred

THERAPEUTIC CLASS:
Glucocorticoid

GENERAL USES:
Endocrine, skin, blood
disorders; asthma

DOSAGE FORMS:
Orally disintegrating
tablets and Tablets:
5 mg; Syrup and Oral
suspension: 5 mg/5 mL,
15 mg/5 mL

PREDNISONE
PRED ni sone

TRADE NAME(S):
Deltasone, Prednicen-M,
Meticorten, Panasol-S

THERAPEUTIC CLASS:
Glucocorticoid

GENERAL USES:
Endocrine, skin, blood
disorders

DOSAGE FORMS:
Tablets: 1 mg, 2.5 mg,
5 mg, 10 mg, 20 mg,
50 mg; Syrup and
Solution: 5 mg/5 mL;
Concentrated solution:
5 mg/mL

PREGABALIN
pre GAB a lin

TRADE NAME(S):
Lyrica

THERAPEUTIC CLASS:
Anticonvulsant, analgesic

GENERAL USES:
Neuropathic pain,
fibromyalgia, seizures

DOSAGE FORMS:
Capsules: 25 mg,
50 mg, 75 mg,
100 mg, 150 mg,
200 mg, 225 mg,
300 mg

PRIMAQUINE
PRIM a kween

TRADE NAME(S):
Primaquine

THERAPEUTIC CLASS:
Antimalarial

GENERAL USES:
Malaria treatment

DOSAGE FORMS:
Tablets: 26.3 mg

PRIMIDONE
PRI mi done

Trade Name(s):
Mysoline

Therapeutic Class:
Anticonvulsant

General Uses:
Seizures

Dosage Forms:
Tablets: 50 mg, 250 mg;
Suspension: 250 mg/
5 mL

PROBENECID
proe BEN e sid

Trade Name(s):
Benemid, Probalan

Therapeutic Class:
Gout agent

General Uses:
Gout

Dosage Forms:
Tablets: 500 mg

PROCAINAMIDE
pro KANE a mide

Trade Name(s):
Pronestyl,
Procanbid

Therapeutic Class:
Antiarrhythmic

General Uses:
Arrhythmias

Dosage Forms:
Tablets: 250 mg, 375 mg,
500 mg; Sustained-
release tablets: 250 mg,
500 mg, 750 mg,
1000 mg; Capsules:
250 mg, 375 mg, 500 mg;
Injection: 1 g

PROCHLORPERAZINE
proe klor PER a zeen

Trade Name(s):
Compazine

Therapeutic Class:
Antiemetic, antipsychotic

General Uses:
Emesis, psychotic
disorders, anxiety

Dosage Forms:
Tablets: 5 mg, 10 mg,
25 mg; Sustained-release
capsules: 10 mg, 15 mg,
30 mg; Syrup: 5 mg/
5 mL; Injection: 10 mg,
50 mg

PROCYCLIDINE
proe SYE kli deen

Trade Name(s):
Kemadrin

Therapeutic Class:
Antiparkinson agent

General Uses:
Parkinson's disease, drug-
induced extrapyramidal
disorders

Dosage Forms:
Tablets: 5 mg

PROGESTERONE
proe JES ter one

Trade Name(s):
Prometrium

THERAPEUTIC CLASS:
Hormone (progesterone)
GENERAL USES:
Amenorrhea, uterine
bleeding
DOSAGE FORMS:
Capsules: 100 mg;
Vaginal gel: 4%, 8%

PROMETHAZINE
proe METH a zeen
TRADE NAME(S):
Phenergan, Promethegan
THERAPEUTIC CLASS:
Antiemetic, antihistamine
GENERAL USES:
Nausea, sedation,
allergies
DOSAGE FORMS:
Tablets and Suppositories:
12.5 mg, 25 mg, 50 mg;
Syrup: 6.25 mg/5 mL;
Injection: 25 mg, 50 mg

PROPAFENONE
proe pa FEEN one
TRADE NAME(S):
Rythmol
THERAPEUTIC CLASS:
Antiarrhythmic
GENERAL USES:
Arrhythmias, tachycardia
DOSAGE FORMS:
Tablets: 150 mg, 225 mg,
300 mg

PROPANTHELINE
proe PAN the leen

TRADE NAME(S):
Pro-Banthine
THERAPEUTIC CLASS:
GI agent
GENERAL USES:
Peptic ulcer
DOSAGE FORMS:
Tablets: 7.5 mg,
15 mg

PROPOXYPHENE
proe POKS i feen
TRADE NAME(S):
Darvon-N, Darvon
THERAPEUTIC CLASS:
Analgesic (narcotic)
GENERAL USES:
Pain
DOSAGE FORMS:
Tablets: 100 mg;
Capsules: 65 mg

PROPOXYPHENE HCL/ACETAMINOPHEN
proe POKS i feen/a seet a
MIN oh fen
TRADE NAME(S):
Wygesic, Balacet
THERAPEUTIC CLASS:
Analgesic
GENERAL USES:
Pain
DOSAGE FORMS:
Tablets: 65 mg/650 mg,
100 mg/325 mg

**PROPOXYPHENE HCL/
ASPIRIN/CAFFEINE**
proe POKS i feen/AS pir
in/ka FEEN
TRADE NAME(S):
Darvon Compound-65
THERAPEUTIC CLASS:
Analgesic
GENERAL USES:
Pain
DOSAGE FORMS:
Pulvules: 65 mg/389 mg/
32.4 mg

**PROPOXYPHENE
NAPSYLATE/
ACETAMINOPHEN**
proe POKS i feen NAP si
late/a seet a MIN oh fen
TRADE NAME(S):
Darvocet N-50, Darvocet
N-100
THERAPEUTIC CLASS:
Analgesic
GENERAL USES:
Pain
DOSAGE FORMS:
Tablets: 50 mg/325 mg,
100 mg/650 mg

PROPRANOLOL
proe PRAN oh lole
TRADE NAME(S):
Inderal, Inderal LA,
Betachron ER, Innopran XL
THERAPEUTIC CLASS:
Cardiac agent,
antimigraine

GENERAL USES:
Hypertension, angina,
MI, migraines, essential
tremor
DOSAGE FORMS:
Tablets: 10 mg, 20 mg,
40 mg, 60 mg, 80 mg,
90 mg; Sustained-release
and Extended-release
capsules: 60 mg,
80 mg, 120 mg, 160 mg;
Solution: 4 mg/mL,
8 mg/mL; Concentrated
solution: 80 mg/mL;
Injection: 1 mg

PROPRANOLOL/HCTZ
proe PRAN oh lole/hye droe
klor oh THYE a zide
TRADE NAME(S):
Inderide, Inderide LA
THERAPEUTIC CLASS:
Antihypertensive/diuretic
GENERAL USES:
Hypertension
DOSAGE FORMS:
Tablets: 40 mg/25 mg,
80 mg/25 mg; Long-
acting capsules: 80 mg/
50 mg, 120 mg/50 mg,
160 mg/50 mg

PROPYLTHIOURACIL
proe pil thye oh YOOR a sil
TRADE NAME(S):
Propylthiouracil
THERAPEUTIC CLASS:
Antithyroid agent

GENERAL USES:
Hyperthyroidism
DOSAGE FORMS:
Tablets: 50 mg

PROTRIPTYLINE
proe TRIP ti leen
TRADE NAME(S):
Vivactil
THERAPEUTIC CLASS:
Antidepressant
GENERAL USES:
Depression
DOSAGE FORMS:
Tablets: 5 mg, 10 mg

PYRAZINAMIDE
peer a ZIN a mide
TRADE NAME(S):
Pyrazinamide
THERAPEUTIC CLASS:
Antituberculosis
agent
GENERAL USES:
Tuberculosis
DOSAGE FORMS:
Tablets: 500 mg

QUAZEPAM
KWAY ze pam
TRADE NAME(S):
Doral
THERAPEUTIC CLASS:
Sedative/hypnotic
GENERAL USES:
Insomnia

DOSAGE FORMS:
Tablets: 7.5 mg,
15 mg

QUETIAPINE
kwe TYE a peen
TRADE NAME(S):
Seroquel, Seroquel XR
THERAPEUTIC CLASS:
Antipsychotic
GENERAL USES:
Psychotic disorders
DOSAGE FORMS:
Tablets: 25 mg, 100 mg,
200 mg, 300 mg;
Extended-release tablets:
200 mg, 300 mg, 400 mg

QUINAPRIL
KWIN a pril
TRADE NAME(S):
Accupril
THERAPEUTIC CLASS:
Antihypertensive, cardiac
agent
GENERAL USES:
Hypertension, heart failure
DOSAGE FORMS:
Tablets: 5 mg, 10 mg,
20 mg, 40 mg

QUINAPRIL/HCTZ
KWIN a pril/hye droe klor oh
THYE a zide
TRADE NAME(S):
Quinaretic, Accuretic
THERAPEUTIC CLASS:
Antihypertensive/
diuretic

GENERAL USES:
Hypertension
DOSAGE FORMS:
Tablets: 10 mg/12.5 mg,
20 mg/12.5 mg, 20 mg/
25 mg

QUINIDINE GLUCONATE
KWIN i deen
TRADE NAME(S):
Quinaglute, Quinalan
THERAPEUTIC CLASS:
Antiarrhythmic
GENERAL USES:
Atrial fibrillation,
tachycardia
DOSAGE FORMS:
Sustained-release tablets:
324 mg; Injection: 800 mg

QUINIDINE SULFATE
KWIN i deen
TRADE NAME(S):
Quinora, Quinidex
Extentabs
THERAPEUTIC CLASS:
Antiarrhythmic
GENERAL USES:
Atrial fibrillation,
tachycardia
DOSAGE FORMS:
Tablets: 200 mg, 300 mg;
Extended-release tablets:
300 mg

QUININE SULFATE
KWYE nine

TRADE NAME(S):
Quinine
THERAPEUTIC CLASS:
Antimalarial
GENERAL USES:
Chloroquine-resistant
malaria
DOSAGE FORMS:
Capsules: 200 mg,
260 mg, 325 mg;
Tablets: 260 mg

RABEPRAZOLE
ra BEP ra zole
TRADE NAME(S):
Aciphex
THERAPEUTIC CLASS:
Gastric acid secretion
inhibitor
GENERAL USES:
GERD, duodenal ulcer,
hyperacidity disorders
DOSAGE FORMS:
Delayed-release tablets:
20 mg

RALOXIFENE
ral OKS i feen
TRADE NAME(S):
Evista
THERAPEUTIC CLASS:
Hormones
(estrogen modulator)
GENERAL USES:
Osteoporosis prevention
DOSAGE FORMS:
Tablets: 60 mg

RALTEGRAVIR POTASSIUM
ral TEG ra vir
Trade Name(s):
Isentress
Therapeutic Class:
Antiviral
General Uses:
HIV infection
Dosage Forms:
Tablets: 400 mg

RAMELTEON
ra MEL tee on
Trade Name(s):
Rozerem
Therapeutic Class:
Sedative/hypnotic
General Uses:
Insomnia
Dosage Forms:
Tablets: 8 mg

RAMIPRIL
RA mi pril
Trade Name(s):
Altace
Therapeutic Class:
Antihypertensive, cardiac agent
General Uses:
Hypertension, CHF
Dosage Forms:
Capsules and Tablets: 1.25 mg, 2.5 mg, 5 mg, 10 mg

RANIBIZUMAB
ra ni BIZ oo mab
Trade Name(s):
Lucentis
Therapeutic Class:
Ocular agent
General Uses:
Wet macular degeneration
Dosage Forms:
Injection: 2 mL

RANITIDINE
ra NI ti deen
Trade Name(s):
Zantac 75, Zantac EFFERdose, Zantac GELdose
Therapeutic Class:
Gastric acid secretion inhibitor
General Uses:
Duodenal ulcer, GERD, heartburn (OTC)
Dosage Forms:
Tablets: 75 mg; Tablets and Capsules: 150 mg, 300 mg; Effervescent tablets/granules: 25 mg, 150 mg; Syrup: 15 mg/ mL; Injection: 50 mg, 150 mg, 1 g

RANOLAZINE
ra NOE la zeen
Trade Name(s):
Ranexa

THERAPEUTIC CLASS:
Antianginal

GENERAL USES:
Chronic angina

DOSAGE FORMS:
Extended-release tablets:
500 mg

RASAGILINE
ra SA ji leen

TRADE NAME(S):
Azilect

THERAPEUTIC CLASS:
Antiparkinson agent

GENERAL USES:
Parkinson's disease

DOSAGE FORMS:
Tablets: 0.5 mg, 1 mg

RASBURICASE
ras BYOOR i kayse

TRADE NAME(S):
Elitek

THERAPEUTIC CLASS:
Antigout

GENERAL USES:
Gout related to
chemotherapy/cancer

DOSAGE FORMS:
Injection: 1.5 mg

REGADENOSON
re ga DEN oh son

TRADE NAME(S):
Lexiscan

THERAPEUTIC CLASS:
Radioimaging enhancer

GENERAL USES:
Cardiac perfusion imaging

DOSAGE FORMS:
Injection: 0.4 mg

REPAGLINIDE
re PAG li nide

TRADE NAME(S):
Prandin

THERAPEUTIC CLASS:
Antidiabetic

GENERAL USES:
Diabetes (type 2)

DOSAGE FORMS:
Tablets: 0.5 mg, 1 mg,
2 mg

REPAGLINIDE/ METFORMIN
re PAG li nide/met FOR min

TRADE NAME(S):
PrandiMet

THERAPEUTIC CLASS:
Antidiabetic

GENERAL USES:
Diabetes (type 2)

DOSAGE FORMS:
Tablets: 1 mg/500 mg,
2 mg/500 mg

RETAPAMULIN
re te PAM ue lin

TRADE NAME(S):
Altabax

THERAPEUTIC CLASS:
Anti-infective (topical)

GENERAL USES:
Impetigo
DOSAGE FORMS:
Ointment: 1%

RETEPLASE
RE ta plase
TRADE NAME(S):
Retavase
THERAPEUTIC CLASS:
Thrombolytic agent
GENERAL USES:
Dissolves blood clots in MI
DOSAGE FORMS:
Injection:
10.8 international units
(18.8 mg)

RIBAVIRIN (AEROSOL)
rye ba VYE rin
TRADE NAME(S):
Virazole
THERAPEUTIC CLASS:
Antiviral
GENERAL USES:
Severe lower respiratory
tract infections in
infants
DOSAGE FORMS:
Aerosol: 6 g

RIBAVIRIN (ORAL)
rye ba VYE rin
TRADE NAME(S):
Rebetrol
THERAPEUTIC CLASS:
Antiviral

GENERAL USES:
Chronic hepatitis C
DOSAGE FORMS:
Capsules: 200 mg

RIFABUTIN
rif a BYOO tin
TRADE NAME(S):
Mycobutin
THERAPEUTIC CLASS:
Antituberculosis
agent
GENERAL USES:
Tuberculosis
DOSAGE FORMS:
Capsules: 150 mg

RIFAMPIN
rif AM pin
TRADE NAME(S):
Rifadin, Rimactane
THERAPEUTIC CLASS:
Antituberculosis agent
GENERAL USES:
Tuberculosis
DOSAGE FORMS:
Capsules: 150 mg,
300 mg; Injection:
600 mg

RIFAPENTINE
rif a PEN teen
TRADE NAME(S):
Priftin
THERAPEUTIC CLASS:
Antituberculosis
agent

General Uses:
Tuberculosis
Dosage Forms:
Tablets: 150 mg

RIFAXIMIN
rif AKS i min
Trade Name(s):
Xifaxan
Therapeutic Class:
Antibacterial
General Uses:
Traveler's diarrhea
Dosage Forms:
Tablets: 200 mg

RILONACEPT
ril ON a sept
Trade Name(s):
Arcalyst
Therapeutic Class:
Interleukin-1 blocker
General Uses:
Cryopyrin-associated
periodic syndromes
(CAPS)
Dosage Forms:
Injection: 160 mg

RILUZOLE
RIL yoo zole
Trade Name(s):
Rilutek
Therapeutic Class:
Amyotrophic lateral
sclerosis agent
General Uses:
Amyotrophic lateral

sclerosis
Dosage Forms:
Tablets: 50 mg

RIMANTADINE
ri MAN ta deen
Trade Name(s):
Flumadine
Therapeutic Class:
Antiviral
General Uses:
Influenza A
Dosage Forms:
Tablets: 100 mg; Syrup:
50 mg/5 mL

RIMEXOLONE
ri MEKS oh lone
Trade Name(s):
Vexol
Therapeutic Class:
Ocular agent
General Uses:
Postoperative
ocular
inflammation
Dosage Forms:
Ophthalmic suspension:
1%

RISEDRONATE
ris ED roe nate
Trade Name(s):
Actonel
Therapeutic Class:
Bisphosphonate
General Uses:
Paget's disease,

osteoporosis

DOSAGE FORMS:
Tablets: 5 mg, 30 mg,
35 mg

RISPERIDONE
ris PER i done
TRADE NAME(S):
Risperdal, Risperdal
Consta
THERAPEUTIC CLASS:
Antipsychotic
GENERAL USES:
Psychotic disorders
DOSAGE FORMS:
Tablets: 0.25 mg, 0.5 mg,
1 mg, 2 mg, 3 mg,
4 mg; Solution: 1 mg/
mL; Injection: 25 mg,
37.5 mg, 50 mg; Orally
disintegrating tablets:
0.5 mg, 1 mg, 3 mg,
4 mg

RITONAVIR
ri TOE na veer
TRADE NAME(S):
Norvir
THERAPEUTIC CLASS:
Antiviral
GENERAL USES:
HIV infection
DOSAGE FORMS:
Capsules: 100 mg;
Solution: 80 mg/mL

RITUXIMAB
ri TUK si mab

TRADE NAME(S):
Rituxan
THERAPEUTIC CLASS:
Monoclonal antibody
GENERAL USES:
Non-Hodgkin's
lymphoma, rheumatoid
arthritis
DOSAGE FORMS:
Injection: 100 mg, 500 mg

RIVASTIGMINE
ri va STIG meen
TRADE NAME(S):
Exelon
THERAPEUTIC CLASS:
Alzheimer's agent
GENERAL USES:
Alzheimer's disease and
dementia
DOSAGE FORMS:
Capsules: 1.5 mg, 3 mg,
4.5 mg, 6 mg; Solution:
2 mg/mL

RIVASTIGMINE (TRANSDERMAL)
ri va STIG meen
TRADE NAME(S):
Exelon
THERAPEUTIC CLASS:
Alzheimer's agent
GENERAL USES:
Alzheimer's disease,
Parkinson's dementia
DOSAGE FORMS:
Release rate (mg/24 hr):
4.6 mg, 9.5 mg

RIZATRIPTAN
rye za TRIP tan
TRADE NAME(S):
Maxalt, Maxalt-MLT
THERAPEUTIC CLASS:
Antimigraine agent
GENERAL USES:
Migraines
DOSAGE FORMS:
Tablets and orally
disintegrating tablets:
5 mg, 10 mg

ROPINIROLE
roe PIN i role
TRADE NAME(S):
Requip, Requip XL
THERAPEUTIC CLASS:
Antiparkinson agent
GENERAL USES:
Parkinson's disease,
restless leg syndrome
DOSAGE FORMS:
Tablets: 0.25 mg, 0.5 mg,
1 mg, 2 mg, 5 mg;
Extended-release tablets:
2 mg, 4 mg, 8 mg

ROSIGLITAZONE
roh si GLI ta zone
TRADE NAME(S):
Avandia
THERAPEUTIC CLASS:
Antidiabetic
GENERAL USES:
Diabetes (type 2)
DOSAGE FORMS:
Tablets: 2 mg, 4 mg, 8 mg

**ROSIGLITAZONE/
GLIMEPIRIDE**
roh si GLI ta zone/GLYE me
pye ride
TRADE NAME(S):
Avandaryl
THERAPEUTIC CLASS:
Antidiabetic
GENERAL USES:
Diabetes
DOSAGE FORMS:
Tablets: 4 mg/1 mg,
4 mg/2 mg,
4 mg/4 mg

**ROSIGLITAZONE/
METFORMIN**
roh si GLI ta zone/met FOR
min
TRADE NAME(S):
Avandamet
THERAPEUTIC CLASS:
Antidiabetic
GENERAL USES:
Diabetes
DOSAGE FORMS:
Tablets: 1 mg/500 mg,
2 mg/500 mg, 4 mg/
500 mg, 2 mg/1000 mg,
4 mg/1000 mg

ROSUVASTATIN
roe soo va STAT in
TRADE NAME(S):
Crestor
THERAPEUTIC CLASS:
Antilipemic

GENERAL USES:
Hyperlipidemia
DOSAGE FORMS:
Tablets: 5 mg, 10 mg,
20 mg, 40 mg

ROTAVIRUS LIVE VACCINE
ROE ta vye rus
TRADE NAME(S):
RotaTeq
THERAPEUTIC CLASS:
Vaccine
GENERAL USES:
Prevention of rotavirus
gastroenteritis
DOSAGE FORMS:
Oral suspension: 2 mL

SACROSIDASE
sak ROE si dase
TRADE NAME(S):
Sucraid
THERAPEUTIC CLASS:
Enzyme replacement
GENERAL USES:
Sucrase-isomaltase
deficiency
DOSAGE FORMS:
Solution:
8500 international units/
mL

SALMETEROL
sal ME te role
TRADE NAME(S):
Serevent, Serevent Diskus

THERAPEUTIC CLASS:
Bronchodilator
GENERAL USES:
Asthma, COPD,
bronchospasm
DOSAGE FORMS:
Aerosol: 25 mcg/
actuation; Inhalation
powder pack:
50 mcg

SALSALATE
SAL sa late
TRADE NAME(S):
Disalcid, Amigesic,
Salsitab
THERAPEUTIC CLASS:
Anti-inflammatory/
analgesic
GENERAL USES:
Pain, osteoarthritis,
rheumatoid arthritis
DOSAGE FORMS:
Capsules: 500 mg; Tablets:
500 mg, 750 mg

SAPROPTERIN
sap roe TER in
TRADE NAME(S):
Kuvan
THERAPEUTIC CLASS:
Enzyme
GENERAL USES:
Reduce blood
phenylalanine
DOSAGE FORMS:
Tablets: 100 mg

SAQUINAVIR
sa KWIN a veer
TRADE NAME(S):
 Invirase
THERAPEUTIC CLASS:
 Antiviral
GENERAL USES:
 HIV infection
DOSAGE FORMS:
 Tablets: 200 mg, 500 mg

SCOPOLAMINE
skoe POL a meen
TRADE NAME(S):
 Transderm-Scop
THERAPEUTIC CLASS:
 Antiemetic/antivertigo
 agent
GENERAL USES:
 Motion sickness
DOSAGE FORMS:
 Transdermal patch:
 1.5 mg

SECOBARBITAL
see koe BAR bi tal
TRADE NAME(S):
 Seconal
THERAPEUTIC CLASS:
 Sedative/hypnotic
GENERAL USES:
 Insomnia (short term
 therapy)
DOSAGE FORMS:
 Capsules: 100 mg

SECRETIN
se KREE tin

TRADE NAME(S):
 SecreFlo
THERAPEUTIC CLASS:
 Diagnostic agent
GENERAL USES:
 Pancreatic dysfunction/
 tumor
DOSAGE FORMS:
 Injection: 16 mcg

SELEGILINE
se LE ji leen
TRADE NAME(S):
 Eldepryl, Zelapar
THERAPEUTIC CLASS:
 Antiparkinson agent
GENERAL USES:
 Parkinson's disease
DOSAGE FORMS:
 Tablets and Capsules:
 5 mg; Orally disintegrating
 tablets: 1.25 mg

**SELEGILINE
(TRANSDERMAL)**
se LE ji leen
TRADE NAME(S):
 Emsam
THERAPEUTIC CLASS:
 CNS agent,
 antidepressant
GENERAL USES:
 Depression
DOSAGE FORMS:
 Patch: 6 mg, 9 mg,
 12 mg

SERTACONAZOLE (TOPICAL)
ser ta KOE na zole

TRADE NAME(S):
Ertaczo

THERAPEUTIC CLASS:
Antifungal

GENERAL USES:
Tinea pedis

DOSAGE FORMS:
Cream: 2%

SERTRALINE
SER tra leen

TRADE NAME(S):
Zoloft

THERAPEUTIC CLASS:
Antidepressant

GENERAL USES:
Depression, OCD, panic disorder, social anxiety, PMDD

DOSAGE FORMS:
Tablets: 25 mg, 50 mg, 100 mg; Concentrated solution: 20 mg/mL

SEVELAMER CARBONATE
se VEL a mer

TRADE NAME(S):
Renvela

THERAPEUTIC CLASS:
Phosphate-binding agent

GENERAL USES:
High phosphorus levels in kidney disease

DOSAGE FORMS:
Tablets: 800 mg

SEVELAMER HCL
se VEL a mer

TRADE NAME(S):
Renagel

THERAPEUTIC CLASS:
Phosphate-binding agent

GENERAL USES:
High phosphorus levels in kidney disease

DOSAGE FORMS:
Tablets: 400 mg, 800 mg

SIBUTRAMINE
si BYOO tra meen

TRADE NAME(S):
Meridia

THERAPEUTIC CLASS:
Anorexiant

GENERAL USES:
Obesity

DOSAGE FORMS:
Capsules: 5 mg, 10 mg, 15 mg

SILDENAFIL
sil DEN a fil

TRADE NAME(S):
Viagra

THERAPEUTIC CLASS:
Impotence agent

GENERAL USES:
Erectile dysfunction

DOSAGE FORMS:
Tablets: 25 mg, 50 mg, 100 mg

SILDENAFIL CITRATE
sil DEN a fil
TRADE NAME(S):
Revatio
THERAPEUTIC CLASS:
Antihypertensive
GENERAL USES:
Pulmonary hypertension
DOSAGE FORMS:
Tablets: 20 mg

SIMVASTATIN
SIM va stat in
TRADE NAME(S):
Zocor
THERAPEUTIC CLASS:
Antilipemic
GENERAL USES:
Hyperlipidemia, CHD
DOSAGE FORMS:
Tablets: 5 mg, 10 mg, 20 mg, 40 mg, 80 mg

SIMVASTATIN/NIACIN
SIM va stat in/NYE a sin
TRADE NAME(S):
Simcor
THERAPEUTIC CLASS:
Antilipemic
GENERAL USES:
Hyperlipidemia
DOSAGE FORMS:
Extended-release tablets: 20 mg/500 mg, 20 mg/

750 mg, 20 mg/1000 mg

SINECATECHINS (TOPICAL)
sin a CAT ah kins
TRADE NAME(S):
Veregen
THERAPEUTIC CLASS:
Dermatologic agent
GENERAL USES:
Genital and perianal warts
DOSAGE FORMS:
Ointment: 15%

SIROLIMUS
sir OH li mus
TRADE NAME(S):
Rapamune
THERAPEUTIC CLASS:
Immunomodulator
GENERAL USES:
Prevent organ transplant rejection
DOSAGE FORMS:
Solution: 1 mg/mL; Tablets: 1 mg

SITAGLIPTIN
sit a GLIP tin
TRADE NAME(S):
Januvia
THERAPEUTIC CLASS:
Antidiabetic
GENERAL USES:
Diabetes
DOSAGE FORMS:
Tablets: 25 mg, 50 mg, 100 mg

SITAGLIPTIN/ METFORMIN
sit a GLIP tin/met FOR min

TRADE NAME(S):
Janumet

THERAPEUTIC CLASS:
Antidiabetic

GENERAL USES:
Diabetes (type 2)

DOSAGE FORMS:
Tablets: 50 mg/500 mg,
50 mg/1000 mg

SODIUM TETRADECYL SULFATE
SO dee um tetra DEK il

TRADE NAME(S):
Sotradecol

THERAPEUTIC CLASS:
Sclerosing agent

GENERAL USES:
Varicose veins

DOSAGE FORMS:
Injection: 1%, 3%

SOLIFENACIN SUCCINATE
sol i FEN a sin

TRADE NAME(S):
VESIcare

THERAPEUTIC CLASS:
Anticholinerigc

GENERAL USES:
Overactive bladder

DOSAGE FORMS:
Tablets: 5 mg, 10 mg

SORAFENIB TOSYLATE
sor AF e nib TOE sil ate

TRADE NAME(S):
Nexavar

THERAPEUTIC CLASS:
Antineoplastic

GENERAL USES:
Advanced renal cell
carcinoma

DOSAGE FORMS:
Tablets: 200 mg

SOTALOL
SOE ta lole

TRADE NAME(S):
Betapace, Betapace
AF

THERAPEUTIC CLASS:
Antiarrhythmic

GENERAL USES:
Arrhythmias

DOSAGE FORMS:
Tablets: 80 mg,
120 mg, 160 mg, 240 mg

SPARFLOXACIN
spar FLOKS a sin

TRADE NAME(S):
Zagam

THERAPEUTIC CLASS:
Anti-infective

GENERAL USES:
Bacterial infections

DOSAGE FORMS:
Tablets: 200 mg

SPIRONOLACTONE
speer on oh LAK tone

TRADE NAME(S):
Aldactone

THERAPEUTIC CLASS:
Diuretic

GENERAL USES:
Edema, hypertension,
hyperaldosteronism

DOSAGE FORMS:
Tablets: 25 mg, 50 mg,
100 mg

STAVUDINE (d4T)
STAV yoo deen

TRADE NAME(S):
Zerit

THERAPEUTIC CLASS:
Antiviral

GENERAL USES:
HIV infection

DOSAGE FORMS:
Capsules: 15 mg, 20 mg,
30 mg, 40 mg; Powder:
1 mg/mL

STREPTOKINASE
strep toe KYE nase

TRADE NAME(S):
Streptase

THERAPEUTIC CLASS:
Thrombolytic agent

GENERAL USES:
Dissolves blood
clots

DOSAGE FORMS:
Injection: 250,000
international units,
750,000 international

units, 1.5 million
international units

SUCRALFATE
soo KRAL fate

TRADE NAME(S):
Carafate

THERAPEUTIC CLASS:
Gastric protectant

GENERAL USES:
Duodenal ulcer

DOSAGE FORMS:
Tablets: 1 g; Suspension:
1 g/10 mL

SULFADIAZINE
sul fa DYE a zeen

TRADE NAME(S):
Microsulfon

THERAPEUTIC CLASS:
Anti-infective

GENERAL USES:
Bacterial infections

DOSAGE FORMS:
Tablets: 500 mg

SULFASALAZINE
sul fa SAL a zeen

TRADE NAME(S):
Azulfidine, Azulfidine EN

THERAPEUTIC CLASS:
GI agent

GENERAL USES:
Ulcerative colitis,
rheumatoid arthritis

DOSAGE FORMS:
Tablets: 500 mg; Delayed-
release tablets: 500 mg

SULFINPYRAZONE
sul fin PEER a zone
TRADE NAME(S):
Anturane
THERAPEUTIC CLASS:
Gout agent
GENERAL USES:
Gouty arthritis
DOSAGE FORMS:
Tablets: 100 mg;
Capsules: 200 mg

SULINDAC
sul IN dak
TRADE NAME(S):
Clinoril
THERAPEUTIC CLASS:
Anti-inflammatory/
analgesic
GENERAL USES:
Various arthritis
conditions, pain
DOSAGE FORMS:
Tablets: 150 mg, 200 mg

SUMATRIPTAN
soo ma TRIP tan
TRADE NAME(S):
Imitrex
THERAPEUTIC CLASS:
Antimigraine
GENERAL USES:
Migraines
DOSAGE FORMS:
Tablets: 25 mg, 50 mg,
100 mg; Nasal spray:
5 mg, 20 mg; Injection:
6 mg

**SUMATRIPTAN/
NAPROXEN**
soo ma TRIP tan/na PROKS
en
TRADE NAME(S):
Treximet
THERAPEUTIC CLASS:
Antimigraine/NSAID
GENERAL USES:
Migraines
DOSAGE FORMS:
Tablets: 85 mg/500 mg

SUNITINIB MALEATE
su NIT i nib
TRADE NAME(S):
Sutent
THERAPEUTIC CLASS:
Antineoplastic
GENERAL USES:
Gastric and renal cancer
DOSAGE FORMS:
Capsules: 12.5 mg,
25 mg, 50 mg

SUPROFEN
soo PRO fen
TRADE NAME(S):
Profenal
THERAPEUTIC CLASS:
Ocular agent
GENERAL USES:
Maintain pupil dilation
during surgery
DOSAGE FORMS:
Ophthalmic solution: 1%

TACRINE
TAK reen
TRADE NAME(S):
Cognex
THERAPEUTIC CLASS:
Alzheimer's agent
GENERAL USES:
Alzheimer's disease
DOSAGE FORMS:
Capsules: 10 mg, 20 mg,
30 mg, 40 mg

TACROLIMUS
ta KROE li mus
TRADE NAME(S):
Prograf
THERAPEUTIC CLASS:
Immunosuppressant
GENERAL USES:
Prevent organ transplant
rejection
DOSAGE FORMS:
Capsules: 1 mg, 5 mg

TADALAFIL
tah DA la fil
TRADE NAME(S):
Cialis
THERAPEUTIC CLASS:
Impotence agent
GENERAL USES:
Erectile dysfunction
DOSAGE FORMS:
Tablets: 5 mg, 10 mg,
20 mg

TAMOXIFEN
ta MOKS i fen
TRADE NAME(S):
Nolvadex, Soltamox
THERAPEUTIC CLASS:
Antiestrogen/
antineoplastic
GENERAL USES:
Breast cancer
DOSAGE FORMS:
Tablets: 10 mg, 20 mg;
Solution: 10 mg/5 mL

TAMSULOSIN
tam SOO loe sin
TRADE NAME(S):
Flomax
THERAPEUTIC CLASS:
Urologic agent
GENERAL USES:
BPH
DOSAGE FORMS:
Capsules: 0.4 mg

TAZAROTENE
taz AR oh teen
TRADE NAME(S):
Tazorac
THERAPEUTIC CLASS:
Retinoid (topical)
GENERAL USES:
Acne, psoriasis
DOSAGE FORMS:
Gel: 0.05%, 0.1%

TELBIVUDINE
tel BI vue deen

TRADE NAME(S):
Tyzeka

THERAPEUTIC CLASS:
Antiviral

GENERAL USES:
Hepatitis B

DOSAGE FORMS:
Tablets: 600 mg

TELITHROMYCIN
tel ITH roe my sin

TRADE NAME(S):
Ketek

THERAPEUTIC CLASS:
Anti-infective

GENERAL USES:
Community-acquired pneumonia, acute bronchitis/sinusitis

DOSAGE FORMS:
Tablets: 400 mg

TELMISARTAN
tel mi SAR tan

TRADE NAME(S):
Micardis

THERAPEUTIC CLASS:
Antihypertensive

GENERAL USES:
Hypertension

DOSAGE FORMS:
Tablets: 40 mg, 80 mg

TEMAZEPAM
te MAZ e pam

TRADE NAME(S):
Restoril

THERAPEUTIC CLASS:
Sedative/hypnotic

GENERAL USES:
Insomnia

DOSAGE FORMS:
Capsules: 7.5 mg, 15 mg, 30 mg

TEMOZOLOMIDE
te moe ZOE loe mide

TRADE NAME(S):
Temodar

THERAPEUTIC CLASS:
Antineoplastic

GENERAL USES:
Astrocytoma (brain tumor)

DOSAGE FORMS:
Capsules: 5 mg, 20 mg, 100 mg, 250 mg

TEMSIROLIMUS
tem sir OH li mus

TRADE NAME(S):
Torisel

THERAPEUTIC CLASS:
Antineoplastic

GENERAL USES:
Kidney cancer

DOSAGE FORMS:
Injection: 10 mg

TENECTEPLASE
ten EK te plase

TRADE NAME(S):
TNKase

THERAPEUTIC CLASS:
Thrombolytic

GENERAL USES:
Dissolves blood clots in MI

DOSAGE FORMS:
Injection: 50 mg

TENOFOVIR
te NOE fo veer

TRADE NAME(S):
Viread

THERAPEUTIC CLASS:
Antiviral

GENERAL USES:
HIV infection

DOSAGE FORMS:
Tablets: 300 mg

TENOFOVIR/ EMTRICITABINE
te NOE fo veer/em trye SYE ta been

TRADE NAME(S):
Truvada

THERAPEUTIC CLASS:
Antiviral

GENERAL USES:
HIV infection

DOSAGE FORMS:
Tablets: 300 mg/200 mg

TERAZOSIN
ter AY zoe sin

TRADE NAME(S):
Terazosin

THERAPEUTIC CLASS:
Antihypertensive, BPH agent

GENERAL USES:
Hypertension, BPH

DOSAGE FORMS:
Capsules, Tablets: 1 mg, 2 mg, 5 mg, 10 mg

TERBINAFINE
TER bin a feen

TRADE NAME(S):
Lamisil

THERAPEUTIC CLASS:
Antifungal

GENERAL USES:
Nail fungal infections, ringworm, athlete's foot

DOSAGE FORMS:
Tablets: 250 mg; Cream and Gel: 1%

TERBUTALINE
ter BYOO ta leen

TRADE NAME(S):
Brethine

THERAPEUTIC CLASS:
Bronchodilator

GENERAL USES:
Bronchospasm, asthma

DOSAGE FORMS:
Tablets: 2.5 mg, 5 mg; Inhaler: 0.2 mg/inhalation; Injection: 1 mg

TERCONAZOLE
ter KONE a zole

TRADE NAME(S):
Terazol-7, Terazol-3

THERAPEUTIC CLASS:
Vaginal antifungal

GENERAL USES:
Vaginal candidiasis
DOSAGE FORMS:
Vaginal cream:
0.4%, 0.8%; Vaginal
suppository: 80 mg

TERIPARATIDE
ter i PAR a tide
TRADE NAME(S):
Forteo
THERAPEUTIC CLASS:
Parathyroid hormone
GENERAL USES:
Osteoporosis in
postmenopause
DOSAGE FORMS:
Injection: 750 mcg

TESTOSTERONE (BUCCAL)
tes TOS ter one
TRADE NAME(S):
Striant
THERAPEUTIC CLASS:
Hormone (testosterone)
GENERAL USES:
Testosterone replacement
DOSAGE FORMS:
Buccal system: 30 mg

TESTOSTERONE (TOPICAL)
tes TOS ter one
TRADE NAME(S):
Androgel, Testim

THERAPEUTIC CLASS:
Hormone (testosterone)
GENERAL USES:
Replacement therapy in
men
DOSAGE FORMS:
Gel: 1%

TESTOSTERONE (TRANSDERMAL)
tes TOS ter one
TRADE NAME(S):
Androderm
THERAPEUTIC CLASS:
Hormone
GENERAL USES:
Replacement therapy in
men
DOSAGE FORMS:
Patch: 2.5 mg/24 hr,
5 mg/24 hr

TETRABENAZINE
tet ra BEN a zeen
TRADE NAME(S):
Xenazine
THERAPEUTIC CLASS:
Monoamine depletor
GENERAL USES:
Chorea in Huntington's
disease
DOSAGE FORMS:
Tablets: 12.5 mg, 25 mg

TETRACYCLINE
tet ra SYE kleen

TRADE NAME(S):
Sumycin, Tetracyn
THERAPEUTIC CLASS:
Anti-infective
GENERAL USES:
Bacterial infections
DOSAGE FORMS:
Capsules and Tablets:
250 mg, 500 mg;
Suspension: 125 mg/
5 mL

THALIDOMIDE
tha LI doe mide
TRADE NAME(S):
Thalomid
THERAPEUTIC CLASS:
Immunomodulator
GENERAL USES:
Erythema nodosum
leprosum (skin disorder),
multiple myeloma
DOSAGE FORMS:
Capsules: 50 mg, 100 mg,
200 mg

THEOPHYLLINE
thee OFF i lin
TRADE NAME(S):
Slo-Phyllin, Theo-Dur,
several others
THERAPEUTIC CLASS:
Bronchodilator
GENERAL USES:
Bronchial asthma,
bronchospasm

DOSAGE FORMS:
Tablets: 100 mg, 125 mg,
200 mg, 250 mg, 300 mg;
Capsules: 100 mg,
200 mg; Syrup and
Elixir: 26.7 mg/5 mL;
Syrup: 50 mg/5 mL;
Timed-release tablets and
capsules: 50 mg, 75 mg,
100 mg, 125 mg, 200 mg,
250 mg, 300 mg, 400 mg,
500 mg, 600 mg

THIOPENTAL
thye oh PEN tal
TRADE NAME(S):
Pentothal
THERAPEUTIC CLASS:
Anesthetic
GENERAL USES:
Anesthesia
DOSAGE FORMS:
Injection: 250 mg,
400 mg, 500 mg, 1 g,
2.5 g, 5 g

THIORIDAZINE
thye oh RID a zeen
TRADE NAME(S):
Mellaril, Mellaril-S
THERAPEUTIC CLASS:
Antipsychotic
GENERAL USES:
Psychotic disorders,
emesis
DOSAGE FORMS:
Tablets: 10 mg, 15 mg,

25 mg, 50 mg, 100 mg,
150 mg, 200 mg;
Concentrated solution:
30 mg/mL, 100 mg/mL;
Suspension: 25 mg/5 mL,
100 mg/5 mL

THIOTHIXENE
thye oh THIKS een
TRADE NAME(S):
Navane
THERAPEUTIC CLASS:
Antipsychotic
GENERAL USES:
Psychotic/behavioral
disorders
DOSAGE FORMS:
Capsules: 1 mg, 2 mg,
5 mg, 10 mg, 20 mg;
Concentrated solution:
5 mg/mL

THYROID DESICCATED
THYE roid DESS i kate ed
TRADE NAME(S):
Armour-Thyroid, Nature-
Throid, Westhroid,
Biothroid
THERAPEUTIC CLASS:
Hormone
GENERAL USES:
Hypothyroidism
DOSAGE FORMS:
Tablets: 15 mg, 30 mg,
32.4 mg, 32.5 mg,
60 mg, 64.8 mg,
65 mg, 90 mg, 120 mg,

129.6 mg, 130 mg,
180 mg, 194.4 mg,
195 mg, 240 mg, 300 mg;
Capsules: 7.5 mg, 15 mg,
30 mg, 60 mg, 90 mg,
120 mg, 150 mg, 180 mg,
240 mg

TIAGABINE
tye AG a been
TRADE NAME(S):
Gabitril
THERAPEUTIC CLASS:
Anticonvulsant
GENERAL USES:
Seizures
DOSAGE FORMS:
Tablets: 4 mg, 12 mg,
16 mg, 20 mg

TICARCILLIN
tye kar SIL in
TRADE NAME(S):
Ticar
THERAPEUTIC CLASS:
Anti-infective
GENERAL USES:
Bacterial infections
DOSAGE FORMS:
Injection: 1 g, 3 g, 6 g,
20 g, 30 g

TICARCILLIN/
CLAVULANATE
POTASSIUM
tye kar SIL in/klav yoo LAN
ate

TRADE NAME(S):
   Timentin
THERAPEUTIC CLASS:
   Anti-infective
GENERAL USES:
   Bacterial infections
DOSAGE FORMS:
   Injection: 3 g/0.1 g

TICLOPIDINE
tye KLOE pi deen
TRADE NAME(S):
   Ticlid
THERAPEUTIC CLASS:
   Antiplatelet agent
GENERAL USES:
   Reduce risk of stroke due
   to clots
DOSAGE FORMS:
   Tablets: 250 mg

TIGECYCLINE
ty ge SYE kleen
TRADE NAME(S):
   Tygacil
THERAPEUTIC CLASS:
   Anti-infective
GENERAL USES:
   Various infections
DOSAGE FORMS:
   Injection: 50 mg

TILUDRONATE
tye LOO droe nate
TRADE NAME(S):
   Skelid

THERAPEUTIC CLASS:
   Bisphosphonate
GENERAL USES:
   Paget's disease
DOSAGE FORMS:
   Tablets: 240 mg

TIMOLOL (OCULAR)
TYE moe lole
TRADE NAME(S):
   Betimol, Timoptic, Istalol
THERAPEUTIC CLASS:
   Ocular agent
GENERAL USES:
   Glaucoma/ocular
   hypertension
DOSAGE FORMS:
   Ophthalmic solution:
   0.25%, 0.5%

TIMOLOL (ORAL)
TYE moe lole
TRADE NAME(S):
   Blocadren
THERAPEUTIC CLASS:
   Antihypertensive, cardiac
   agent, anti-migraine agent
GENERAL USES:
   Hypertension, MI,
   migraines
DOSAGE FORMS:
   Tablets: 5 mg, 10 mg,
   20 mg

TIMOLOL/HCTZ
TYE moe lole/hye droe klor
oh THYE a zide

Trade Name(s):
Timolide

Therapeutic Class:
Antihypertensive/
diuretic

General Uses:
Hypertension

Dosage Forms:
Tablets: 10 mg/25 mg

TINIDAZOLE
ty NI da zole

Trade Name(s):
Tindamax

Therapeutic Class:
Antifungal

General Uses:
Antiprotozoal

Dosage Forms:
Tablets: 250 mg, 500 mg

TINZAPARIN
tin ZA pa rin

Trade Name(s):
Innohep

Therapeutic Class:
Anticoagulant (LMWH)

General Uses:
Treatment for deep vein
thrombosis

Dosage Forms:
Injection:
40,000 international units

TIOTROPIUM
ty oh TROE pee um

Trade Name(s):
Spiriva

Therapeutic Class:
Bronchodilator

General Uses:
COPD

Dosage Forms:
Inhaler capsules: 18 mcg

TIPRANAVIR
tip RA na veer

Trade Name(s):
Aptivus

Therapeutic Class:
Antiviral

General Uses:
HIV infection

Dosage Forms:
Capsules: 250 mg; Oral
solution: 100 mg/mL

TIZANIDINE
tye ZAN i deen

Trade Name(s):
Zanaflex

Therapeutic Class:
Skeletal muscle relaxant

General Uses:
Muscle spasticity

Dosage Forms:
Tablets: 4 mg

TOBRAMYCIN (OCULAR)
toe bra MYE sin

Trade Name(s):
Tobrex, AKTob

Therapeutic Class:
Ocular agent (anti-
infective)

GENERAL USES:
Ocular infections

DOSAGE FORMS:
Ophthalmic solution:
0.3%; Ophthalmic
ointment: 3 mg/g

TOBRAMYCIN SULFATE
toe bra MYE sin

TRADE NAME(S):
Nebcin

THERAPEUTIC CLASS:
Anti-infective

GENERAL USES:
Bacterial infections

DOSAGE FORMS:
Injection: 20 mg, 60 mg,
80 mg, 1.2 g; Nebulizer
solution: 300 mg

TOBRAMYCIN/ DEXAMETHASONE (OCULAR)
toe bra MYE sin/deks a
METH a sone

TRADE NAME(S):
TobraDex

THERAPEUTIC CLASS:
Anti-infective/anti-
inflammatory (ocular)

GENERAL USES:
Ocular infection/
inflammation

DOSAGE FORMS:
Ophthalmic
suspension: 0.3%/0.1%;
Ophthalmic ointment:
0.3%/0.1%

TOCAINIDE
toe KAY nide

TRADE NAME(S):
Tonocard

THERAPEUTIC CLASS:
Antiarrhythmic

GENERAL USES:
Ventricular arrhythmias

DOSAGE FORMS:
Tablets: 400 mg, 600 mg

TOLAZAMIDE
tole AZ a mide

TRADE NAME(S):
Tolinase

THERAPEUTIC CLASS:
Antidiabetic

GENERAL USES:
Diabetes (type 2)

DOSAGE FORMS:
Tablets: 100 mg, 250 mg,
500 mg

TOLBUTAMIDE
tole BYOO ta mide

TRADE NAME(S):
Orinase

THERAPEUTIC CLASS:
Antidiabetic

GENERAL USES:
Diabetes (type 2)

DOSAGE FORMS:
Tablets: 500 mg

TOLCAPONE
TOLE ka pone

TRADE NAME(S):
Tasmar

THERAPEUTIC CLASS:
Antiparkinson agent
GENERAL USES:
Parkinson's
disease
DOSAGE FORMS:
Tablets: 100 mg, 200 mg

TOLMETIN
TOLE met in
TRADE NAME(S):
Tolectin
THERAPEUTIC CLASS:
Anti-inflammatory/
analgesic
GENERAL USES:
Osteoarthritis, rheumatoid
arthritis
DOSAGE FORMS:
Tablets: 200 mg, 600 mg;
Capsules: 400 mg

TOLTERODINE
tole TER oh deen
TRADE NAME(S):
Detrol, Detrol LA
THERAPEUTIC CLASS:
Antispasmodic
GENERAL USES:
Bladder instability
DOSAGE FORMS:
Tablets: 1 mg, 2 mg;
Extended-release
capsules: 2 mg, 4 mg

TOPIRAMATE
toe PYRE a mate

TRADE NAME(S):
Topamax
THERAPEUTIC CLASS:
Anticonvulsant
GENERAL USES:
Seizures
DOSAGE FORMS:
Tablets: 25 mg, 100 mg,
200 mg; Sprinkle
capsules: 15 mg, 25 mg

TOREMIFENE
tore EM i feen
TRADE NAME(S):
Fareston
THERAPEUTIC CLASS:
Antiestrogen/
antineoplastic
GENERAL USES:
Breast cancer
DOSAGE FORMS:
Tablets: 60 mg

TORSEMIDE
TORE se mide
TRADE NAME(S):
Demadex
THERAPEUTIC CLASS:
Diuretic
GENERAL USES:
CHF-related edema,
hypertension
DOSAGE FORMS:
Tablets: 5 mg, 10 mg,
20 mg, 100 mg

**TOSITUMOMAB/
IODINE I 131
TOSITUMOMAB**
toe si TYOO mo mab
TRADE NAME(S):
  Bexxar
THERAPEUTIC CLASS:
  Antineoplastic
GENERAL USES:
  Non-Hodgkin's lymphoma
DOSAGE FORMS:
  Injection: 35 mg, 225 mg

TRAMADOL
TRA ma dole
TRADE NAME(S):
  Ultram, Ultram ER
THERAPEUTIC CLASS:
  Analgesic
GENERAL USES:
  Pain
DOSAGE FORMS:
  Tablets: 50 mg; Extended-
  release tablets: 100 mg,
  200 mg, 300 mg

**TRAMADOL/
ACETAMINOPHEN**
TRA ma dole/a seet a MIN
oh fen
TRADE NAME(S):
  Ultracet
THERAPEUTIC CLASS:
  Analgesic
GENERAL USES:
  Short-term treatment of
  pain

DOSAGE FORMS:
  Tablets: 37.5 mg/325 mg

TRANDOLAPRIL
tran DOE la pril
TRADE NAME(S):
  Mavik
THERAPEUTIC CLASS:
  Antihypertensive, cardiac
  agent
GENERAL USES:
  Hypertension, CHF
DOSAGE FORMS:
  Tablets: 1 mg, 2 mg, 4 mg

**TRANDOLAPRIL/
VERAPAMIL**
tran DOE la pril/ver AP a mil
TRADE NAME(S):
  Tarka
THERAPEUTIC CLASS:
  Antihypertensive/diuretic
GENERAL USES:
  Hypertension
DOSAGE FORMS:
  Tablets: 1 mg/240 mg,
  2 mg/240 mg, 4 mg/
  240 mg

TRANYLCYPROMINE
tran il SIP roe meen
TRADE NAME(S):
  Parnate
THERAPEUTIC CLASS:
  Antidepressant
GENERAL USES:
  Depression

DOSAGE FORMS:
Tablets: 10 mg

TRAVOPROST
TRA voe prost
TRADE NAME(S):
Travatan Z
THERAPEUTIC CLASS:
Ocular agent
GENERAL USES:
Open-angle
glaucoma, ocular
hypertension
DOSAGE FORMS:
Ophthalmic solution:
0.004%

TRAZODONE
TRAZ oh done
TRADE NAME(S):
Trazodone
THERAPEUTIC CLASS:
Antidepressant
GENERAL USES:
Depression
DOSAGE FORMS:
Tablets: 50 mg,
100 mg, 150 mg, 300 mg

TREPROSTINIL SODIUM
tre PROST in nil
TRADE NAME(S):
Remodulin
THERAPEUTIC CLASS:
Cardiac agent
GENERAL USES:
Pulmonary arterial
hypertension

DOSAGE FORMS:
Injection: 1 mg, 2.5 mg,
5 mg, 10 mg

TRETINOIN (TOPICAL)
TRET i noyn
TRADE NAME(S):
Retin-A, Retin-A Micro
THERAPEUTIC CLASS:
Retinoid (topical)
GENERAL USES:
Acne vulgaris
DOSAGE FORMS:
Cream and Gel: 0.025%,
0.1%; Cream: 0.05%;
Liquid: 0.05%; Gel:
0.01%

**TRIAMCINOLONE
(INHALED)**
trye am SIN oh lone
TRADE NAME(S):
Azmacort
THERAPEUTIC CLASS:
Corticosteroid (inhaler)
GENERAL USES:
Asthma (chronic)
DOSAGE FORMS:
Inhaler: 100 mcg/
inhalation

**TRIAMCINOLONE
(NASAL)**
trye am SIN oh lone
TRADE NAME(S):
Nasacort, Nasacort
AQ

THERAPEUTIC CLASS:
Corticosteroid (nasal)

GENERAL USES:
Allergies

DOSAGE FORMS:
Nasal spray and Inhaler:
55 mcg/spray

**TRIAMCINOLONE
(ORAL)**
trye am SIN oh lone

TRADE NAME(S):
Kenacort, Aristocort

THERAPEUTIC CLASS:
Glucocorticoid

GENERAL USES:
Endocrine, skin, blood
disorders

DOSAGE FORMS:
Tablets: 4 mg, 8 mg;
Syrup: 4 mg/5 mL

**TRIAMCINOLONE
ACETONIDE**
trye am SIN oh lone

TRADE NAME(S):
Aristocort, Kenalog, Flutex

THERAPEUTIC CLASS:
Corticosteroid (topical)

GENERAL USES:
Various skin conditions

DOSAGE FORMS:
Ointment and Cream:
0.025%, 0.1%, 0.5%;
Lotion: 0.025%, 0.1%

TRIAMTERENE
trye AM ter een

TRADE NAME(S):
Dyrenium

THERAPEUTIC CLASS:
Diuretic

GENERAL USES:
CHF-related edema,
hypertension

DOSAGE FORMS:
Tablets: 50 mg, 100 mg

TRIAZOLAM
trye AY zoe lam

TRADE NAME(S):
Halcion

THERAPEUTIC CLASS:
Sedative/hypnotic

GENERAL USES:
Insomnia

DOSAGE FORMS:
Tablets: 0.125 mg,
0.25 mg

TRIFLUOPERAZINE
trye floo oh PER a zeen

TRADE NAME(S):
Stelazine

THERAPEUTIC CLASS:
Antipsychotic

GENERAL USES:
Psychotic disorders,
anxiety

DOSAGE FORMS:
Tablets: 1 mg, 2 mg, 5 mg,
10 mg; Concentrated
solution: 10 mg/mL;
Injection: 20 mg

TRIFLURIDINE
trye FLURE i deen
TRADE NAME(S):
    Viroptic
THERAPEUTIC CLASS:
    Ocular agent (antiviral)
GENERAL USES:
    Ocular herpes infections
DOSAGE FORMS:
    Ophthalmic
    solution: 1%

TRIHEXYPHENIDYL
trye heks ee FEN i dil
TRADE NAME(S):
    Artane
THERAPEUTIC CLASS:
    Antiparkinson agent
GENERAL USES:
    Parkinson's disease, drug-
    induced extrapyramidal
    disorders
DOSAGE FORMS:
    Tablets: 2 mg, 5 mg;
    Sustained-release
    capsules: 5 mg; Elixir:
    2 mg/5 mL

**TRIMETHOPRIM/
SULFAMETHOXAZOLE**
trye METH oh prim/sul fa
meth OKS a zole
TRADE NAME(S):
    Bactrim, Cotrim,
    Septra
THERAPEUTIC CLASS:
    Anti-infective

GENERAL USES:
    Bacterial infections
DOSAGE FORMS:
    Tablets: 80 mg/400 mg,
    160 mg/800 mg;
    Suspension: 40 mg/
    200 mg/5 mL; Injection:
    800 mg/160 mg,
    1600 mg/320 mg

TRIMIPRAMINE
trye MI pra meen
TRADE NAME(S):
    Surmontil
THERAPEUTIC CLASS:
    Antidepressant
GENERAL USES:
    Depression
DOSAGE FORMS:
    Capsules: 25 mg, 50 mg,
    100 mg

TRIPTORELIN PAMOATE
trip toe REL in
TRADE NAME(S):
    Trelstar Depot, Trelstar LA
THERAPEUTIC CLASS:
    Antineoplastic
GENERAL USES:
    Palliative treatment of
    advanced prostate cancer
DOSAGE FORMS:
    Injection: 3.75 mg,
    11.25 mg

TROLEANDOMYCIN
troe lee an doe MYE sin

TRADE NAME(S):
TAO

THERAPEUTIC CLASS:
Anti-infective

GENERAL USES:
Bacterial infections

DOSAGE FORMS:
Capsules: 250 mg

TROSPIUM
TROSE pee um

TRADE NAME(S):
Sanctura, Sanctura XR

THERAPEUTIC CLASS:
Antispasmodic

GENERAL USES:
Overactive bladder

DOSAGE FORMS:
Tablets: 20 mg; Extended-release capsules: 60 mg

TRYPAN BLUE
TRYE pan

TRADE NAME(S):
Vision Blue

THERAPEUTIC CLASS:
Ocular agent

GENERAL USES:
Cataract surgery

DOSAGE FORMS:
Ophthalmic solution: 0.06%

UNOPROSTONE ISOPROPYL
yoo noe PROS tone

TRADE NAME(S):
Rescula

THERAPEUTIC CLASS:
Ocular agent

GENERAL USES:
Open-angle glaucoma

DOSAGE FORMS:
Ophthalmic solution: 0.15%

URSODIOL
ur soe DYE ole

TRADE NAME(S):
Actigall, Urso

THERAPEUTIC CLASS:
Gallstone solubilizer

GENERAL USES:
Gallstones

DOSAGE FORMS:
Capsules: 300 mg; Tablets: 250 mg, 500 mg

VALACYCLOVIR
val ay SYE kloe veer

TRADE NAME(S):
Valtrex

THERAPEUTIC CLASS:
Antiviral

GENERAL USES:
Herpes, shingles, cold sores, CMV disease

DOSAGE FORMS:
Tablets: 500 mg, 1000 mg

VALGANCICLOVIR
val gan SYE kloh veer

TRADE NAME(S):
Valcyte

THERAPEUTIC CLASS:
Antiviral
GENERAL USES:
CMV retinitis in HIV patients
DOSAGE FORMS:
Tablets: 450 mg

VALPROIC ACID AND DERIVATIVES
val PROE ik AS id
TRADE NAME(S):
Depakote, Depakote ER, Depakene
THERAPEUTIC CLASS:
Anticonvulsant
GENERAL USES:
Seizures
DOSAGE FORMS:
Capsules: 250 mg; Delayed-release tablets: 125 mg, 250 mg, 500 mg; Extended-release tablets: 250 mg, 500 mg; Sprinkle capsules: 125 mg; Syrup: 250 mg/5 mL; Injection: 500 mg

VALSARTAN
val SAR tan
TRADE NAME(S):
Diovan
THERAPEUTIC CLASS:
Antihypertensive
GENERAL USES:
Hypertension, CHF

DOSAGE FORMS:
Capsules: 80 mg, 160 mg, 320 mg

VALSARTAN/HCTZ
val SAR tan/hye droe klor oh THYE a zide
TRADE NAME(S):
Diovan HCT
THERAPEUTIC CLASS:
Antihypertensive/ diuretic
GENERAL USES:
Hypertension
DOSAGE FORMS:
Tablets: 80 mg/ 12.5 mg, 160 mg/12.5 mg, 320 mg/12.5 mg, 320 mg/25 mg

VANCOMYCIN
van koe MYE sin
TRADE NAME(S):
Vancocin, Vancoled
THERAPEUTIC CLASS:
Anti-infective
GENERAL USES:
Bacterial infections
DOSAGE FORMS:
Capsules: 125 mg, 250 mg; Solution: 1 g, 10 g; Injection: 500 mg, 1 g, 2 g, 5 g, 10 g

VARDENAFIL
var DEN a fil
TRADE NAME(S):
Levitra

THERAPEUTIC CLASS:
Impotence agent
GENERAL USES:
Erectile dysfunction
DOSAGE FORMS:
Tablets: 2.5 mg, 5 mg,
10 mg, 20 mg

VARENICLINE
var e NI kleen
TRADE NAME(S):
Chantix
THERAPEUTIC CLASS:
Nicotine agonist
GENERAL USES:
Smoking cessation
DOSAGE FORMS:
Tablets: 0.5 mg, 1 mg

VECURONIUM
ve kyoo ROE ni um
TRADE NAME(S):
Norcuron
THERAPEUTIC CLASS:
Muscle relaxant
GENERAL USES:
Aid to anesthesia
DOSAGE FORMS:
Injection: 10 mg,
20 mg

VENLAFAXINE
ven la FAKS een
TRADE NAME(S):
Effexor, Effexor XR
THERAPEUTIC CLASS:
Antidepressant

GENERAL USES:
Depression, social anxiety
disorder, panic disorder
DOSAGE FORMS:
Tablets: 25 mg, 37.5 mg,
50 mg, 75 mg, 100 mg;
Extended-release tablets:
37.5 mg, 75 mg, 150 mg

VERAPAMIL
ver AP a mil
TRADE NAME(S):
Calan, Isoptin, Verelan,
Isoptin SR, Calan SR,
Verelan PM
THERAPEUTIC CLASS:
Antihypertensive (SR),
antianginal
GENERAL USES:
Hypertension, angina
DOSAGE FORMS:
Tablets: 40 mg, 80 mg,
120 mg; Sustained-
release tablets and
Capsules: 120 mg,
180 mg, 240 mg;
Sustained-release
capsules: 100 mg,
200 mg, 300 mg;
Injection: 5 mg

VIDARABINE
vye DARE a been
TRADE NAME(S):
Vira-A
THERAPEUTIC CLASS:
Ocular agent (antiviral)

General Uses:
Ocular herpes infections

Dosage Forms:
Ophthalmic ointment: 3%

VINBLASTINE
vin BLAS teen

Trade Name(s):
Velban

Therapeutic Class:
Antineoplastic

General Uses:
Various cancers

Dosage Forms:
Injection: 10 mg, 25 mg

VINCRISTINE
vin KRIS teen

Trade Name(s):
Vincasar PFS

Therapeutic Class:
Antineoplastic

General Uses:
Various cancers

Dosage Forms:
Injection: 1 mg, 2 mg, 5 mg

VINORELBINE
vi NOR el been

Trade Name(s):
Navelbine

Therapeutic Class:
Antineoplastic

General Uses:
Various cancers

Dosage Forms:
Injection: 10 mg, 50 mg

VITAMIN K (PHYTONADIONE)
fye toe na DYE one

Trade Name(s):
Aqua-Mephyton, Mephyton

Therapeutic Class:
Vitamin

General Uses:
Blood-clotting disorders

Dosage Forms:
Tablets: 5 mg; Injection: 1 mg

VORICONAZOLE
vor i KOE na zole

Trade Name(s):
VFEND

Therapeutic Class:
Antifungal

General Uses:
Serious fungal infections

Dosage Forms:
Tablets: 50 mg, 200 mg; Injection: 200 mg

VORINOSTAT
vor IN oh stat

Trade Name(s):
Zolinza

Therapeutic Class:
Enzyme inhibitor

General Uses:
Cutaneous T-cell lymphoma

Dosage Forms:
Capsules: 100 mg

WARFARIN
WAR far in

Trade Name(s):
Coumadin

Therapeutic Class:
Anticoagulant

General Uses:
Preventive therapy for blood clots

Dosage Forms:
Tablets: 1 mg, 2 mg, 2.5 mg, 3 mg, 4 mg, 5 mg, 6 mg, 7.5 mg, 10 mg

ZAFIRLUKAST
za FIR loo kast

Trade Name(s):
Accolate

Therapeutic Class:
Bronchodilator

General Uses:
Asthma prevention and treatment

Dosage Forms:
Tablets: 10 mg, 20 mg

ZALEPLON
ZAL e plon

Trade Name(s):
Sonata

Therapeutic Class:
Hypnotic/sedative

General Uses:
Insomnia

Dosage Forms:
Capsules: 5 mg, 10 mg

ZANAMIVIR
za NA mi veer

Trade Name(s):
Relenza

Therapeutic Class:
Antiviral

General Uses:
Influenza A and B

Dosage Forms:
Inhalation: 5 mg/ inhalation

ZICONOTIDE
zi KOE no tide

Trade Name(s):
Prialt

Therapeutic Class:
Analgesic

General Uses:
Severe chronic pain

Dosage Forms:
Injection: 100 mcg, 200 mcg, 500 mcg

ZIDOVUDINE
zye DOE vyoo deen

Trade Name(s):
Retrovir

General Uses:
HIV infection

Dosage Forms:
Capsules: 100 mg;
Tablets: 300 mg; Syrup:
50 mg/mL; Injection:
200 mg

ZILEUTON
zye LOO ton

Trade Name(s):
Zyflo CR

Therapeutic Class:
Antiasthmatic

General Uses:
Asthma prevention and
treatment

Dosage Forms:
Extended-release tablets:
600 mg

ZIPRASIDONE
zi PRAS i done

Trade Name(s):
Geodon

Therapeutic Class:
Antipsychotic

General Uses:
Schizophrenia, bipolar
mania

Dosage Forms:
Capsules: 20 mg, 40 mg,
60 mg, 80 mg; Injection:
20 mg

ZOLEDRONIC ACID
zoe le DRON ik AS id

Trade Name(s):
Zometa, Reclast

Therapeutic Class:
Bisphosphonate

General Uses:
Treatment of
hypercalcemia of cancer,
osteoporosis, Paget's
disease

Dosage Forms:
Injection: 4 mg, 5 mg

ZOLMITRIPTAN
zohl mi TRIP tan

Trade Name(s):
Zomig, Zomig-ZMT

Therapeutic Class:
Antimigraine

General Uses:
Migraines

Dosage Forms:
Tablets: 2.5 mg, 5 mg;
Orally disintegrating
tablets: 2.5 mg, 5 mg;
Nasal spray: 5 mg/0.1 mL

ZOLPIDEM
zole PI dem

Trade Name(s):
Ambien, Ambien CR

Therapeutic Class:
Sedative, hypnotic

General Uses:
Insomnia

DOSAGE FORMS:
 Tablets: 5 mg, 10 mg;
 Extended-release tablets:
 6.25 mg, 12.5 mg

ZONISAMIDE
zoe NIS a mide
TRADE NAME(S):
 Zonegran
THERAPEUTIC CLASS:
 Anticonvulsant
GENERAL USES:
 Partial seizures (adults)
DOSAGE FORMS:
 Capsules: 25 mg, 50 mg,
 100 mg

ZOSTER VACCINE
ZOS ter vak SEEN
TRADE NAME(S):
 Zostavax
THERAPEUTIC CLASS:
 Vaccine
GENERAL USES:
 Prevention of herpes
 zoster (shingles)
DOSAGE FORMS:
 Injection: 0.6

Generic Name	Brand Name(s)	General Use(s)
Acyclovir	Zovirax, Zovirax topical	Herpes simplex and zoster infections
Adapalene	Differin	Acne
Albuterol (aerosol)	Proventil HFA	Bronchospasm
Alendronate	Fosamax	Osteoporosis, Paget's disease
Alteplase	Activase	Dissolves blood clots in MI, stroke, pulmonary embolism, catheter occlusion
Amlodipine	Norvasc	Angina, hypertension
Amlodipine/atorvastatin	Caduet	Hypertension, hyperlipidemia, angina
Amlodipine/benazepril	Lotrel	Hypertension, CHF
Amoxicillin	Amoxil	Bacterial infections
Amphotericin B, lipid based	AmBisome	Systemic fungal infections
Anastrozole	Arimidex	Breast cancer
Aripiprazole	Abilify	Psychotic disorders
Atomoxetine	Strattera	ADHD

Atorvastatin	Lipitor	Hyperlipidemia, hypertriglyceridemia, reduce stroke or MI risk
Azelastine (nasal spray)	Astelin	Allergies
Azithromycin	Zithromax	Bacterial infections
Benzoyl peroxide/clindamycin	BenzaClin	Acne
Bevacizumab	Avastin	Metastatic colorectal cancer
Bimatoprost (ophthalmic solution)	Lumigan	Ocular hypertension, open-angle glaucoma
Bivalirudin	Angiomax	Prevention of clotting in angina/PTCA
Brimonidine (ophthalmic solution)	Alphagan P	Glaucoma/ocular hypertension
Budesonide	Pulmicort Respules	Asthma (chronic)
Budesonide (nasal spray)	Rhinocort Aqua	Allergies
Bupropion (extended/sustained release)	Wellbutrin XL, Budeprion SR	Depression, seasonal affective disorder
Candesartan	Atacand	Hypertension, CHF
Carvedilol	Coreg, Coreg CR	Hypertension, CHF
Cefazolin	Ancef, Kefzol	Bacterial infections

Cefdinir	Omnicef	Bacterial infections
Cefepime	Maxipime	Bacterial infections
Ceftriaxone	Rocephin, ceftriaxone	Bacterial infections
Celecoxib	Celebrex	Osteoarthritis, rheumatoid arthritis, acute pain, dysmenorrhea, FAP
Cetirizine	Zyrtec	Allergic rhinitis, hives
Cetirizine/pseudoephedrine (extended release)	Zyrtec-D	Allergies
Cetuximab	Erbitux	Various cancers
Ciprofloxacin/dexamethasone (otic)	Ciprodex	Acute otitis media
Clarithromycin (extended release)	Biaxin XL	Bacterial infections
Clonidine (transdermal)	Catapres-TTS	Hypertension
Clopidogrel	Plavix	Reduce stroke, MI risk, acute coronary syndrome
Cyclosporine (ocular)	Restasis	Increase tear production
Daptomycin	Cubicin	Bacterial infections

Top 200 Drugs (continued)

Darbepoetin alfa	Aranesp	Anemia
Desloratadine	Clarinex	Allergic rhinitis, chronic urticaria
Dexmethylphenidate	Focalin XR	ADHD
Dextroamphetamine/amphetamine (extended release)	Adderall XR	ADHD
Diclofenac/misoprostol	Arthrotec	Arthritis
Digoxin	Digitek, Lanoxin	CHF, atrial fibrillation
Diltiazem	Tiazac, Taztia XT	Hypertension, angina
Donepezil	Aricept	Alzheimer's disease
Dorzolamide/timolol	Cosopt	Glaucoma/ocular hypertension
Drotrecogin alfa	Xigris	Sepsis
Dutasteride	Avodart	BPH
Eletriptan	Relpax	Migraines
Enoxaparin sodium	Lovenox	Prevention of blood clots
Epoetin alfa	Epogen, Procrit	Anemia

Top 200 Drugs (continued)

Escitalopram	Lexapro	Depression, anxiety
Esomeprazole	Nexium	GERD, erosive esophagitis, Zollinger-Ellison syndrome
Estradiol (transdermal)	Vivelle-Dot, Climara	Estrogen replacement
Estrogens, conjugated	Premarin, Cenestin	Estrogen replacement
Estrogens conjugated/ medroxyprogesterone	Prempro	Estrogen replacement
Eszopiclone	Lunesta	Insomnia
Etanercept	Enbrel	Rheumatoid/psoriatic arthritis, plaque psoriasis, ankylosing spondylitis
Ethinyl estradiol/desogestrel	Apri, Mircette, Kariva	Contraception
Ethinyl estradiol/drospirenone	Yasmin	Contraception
Ethinyl estradiol/ethynodiol	Zovia 1/35E	Contraception
Ethinyl estradiol/etonogestrel	NuvaRing	Contraception
Ethinyl estradiol/levonorgestrel	Aviane, Alesse, Levora, Triphasil, Trivora-28	Contraception

Ethinyl estradiol/norelgestromin (transdermal)	Ortho Evra	Contraception
Ethinyl estradiol/norethindrone	Ortho Novum 7/7/7, Neocon 1/35, Ovcon 35, Estrostep	Contraception
Ethinyl estradiol/norgestimate	Sprintec, Ortho-Cyclen, Ortho-Tri-Cyclen	Contraception
Exenatide	Byetta	Diabetes
Ezetimibe	Zetia	Hyperlipidemia
Ezetimibe/simvastatin	Vytorin	Hypercholesterolemia
Fenofibrate	TriCor	Hyperlipidemia
Fentanyl (transdermal)	Duragesic	Pain
Fexofenadine/pseudoephedrine (extended release)	Allegra-D 12 Hour, Allegra-D 24 Hour	Allergic rhinitis
Finasteride	Proscar, Propecia	BPH, male pattern baldness
Fluoxetine	Prozac	Depression, bulimia, OCD, PMDD
Fluticasone (inhaler)	Flovent HFA	Asthma

Fluticasone/salmeterol (inhaler)	Advair Diskus	Asthma (chronic), COPD
Fluvastatin (extended release)	Lescol XL	Hyperlipidemia, secondary prevention of CHD
Gabapentin	Neurontin	Seizures, postherpetic neuralgia
Gatifloxacin (ocular)	Zymar	Ocular infections
Glimeperide	Amaryl	Diabetes type 2
Glipizide (extended release)	Glucotrol XL, Glipizide ER	Diabetes type 2
Human papillomavirus vaccine	Gardasil	Prevention of diseases caused by HPV in females
Hydrocodone/chlorpheniramine	Tussionex	Cough and cold
Ibandronate	Boniva	Postmenopausal osteoporosis
Imipenem/cilastatin	Primaxin	Bacterial infections
Imiquimod	Aldara	Actinic keratosis, genital and anal warts, basal cell carcinoma
Infliximab	Remicade	Crohn's disease, arthritis syndromes, ulcerative colitis, psoriasis, psoriatic arthritis
Insulin, glargine	Lantus	Diabetes

Insulin, lispro protamine suspension and insulin lispro	Humalog 75/25	Diabetes
Insulin, isophane suspension	Humulin N	Diabetes
Insulin, isophane suspension and insulin regular	Humulin 70/30	Diabetes
Ipratropium/albuterol (inhaler)	Combivent	Bronchospasm
Irbesartan	Avapro	Hypertension, diabetic nephropathy
Irbesartan/HCTZ	Avalide	Hypertension
Ketotifen	Zaditor	Allergic conjunctivitis
Lamotrigine	Lamictal	Seizures, bipolar disorder
Lansoprazole	Prevacid	GERD, duodenal ulcer
Latanoprost (ophthalmic solution)	Xalatan	Glaucoma, ocular hypertension
Lenalidomide	Revlimid	Myelodysplastic syndrome
Levalbuterol (inhalational)	Xopenox, Xopenox HFA	Bronchospasm
Levetiracetam	Keppra	Partial seizures

Levofloxacin	Levaquin	Bacterial infections
Levothyroxine	Synthroid, Levoxyl, Levothroid	Hypothyroidism
Lidocaine (transdermal)	Lidoderm	Postherpetic neuralgia
Linezolid	Zyvox	Vancomycin-resistant bacterial infections
Losartan	Cozaar	Hypertension, diabetic nephropathy
Losartan/HCTZ	Hyzaar	Hypertension
Memantine	Namenda	Alzheimer's disease
Mesalamine	Asacol	Inflammatory bowel disease
Metaxalone	Skelaxin	Musculoskeletal conditions
Metformin/glipizide	Metaglip	Diabetes
Methotrexate	Rheumatrex, Trexall	Cancer, rheumatoid arthritis
Methylphenidate	Concerta, Methylin	ADHD, narcolepsy
Metoclopramide	Reglan, Clopra, Reclomide	Nausea, vomiting
Metoprolol (extended release)	Toprol-XL	Hypertension, angina, MI

Mirtazapine	Remeron	Depression
Modafinil	Provigil	Narcolepsy, sleep disorders
Mometasone (nasal)	Nasonex	Allergies
Montelukast	Singulair	Asthma, seasonal allergies
Morphine sulfate	Morphine sulfate	Pain
Moxifloxacin	Avelox	Bacterial infections
Moxifloxacin (ocular)	Vigamox	Bacterial conjunctivitis
Mupirocin (topical)	Bactroban	Impetigo, skin infection
Niacin	Niaspan	Hyperlipidemia
Nicardipine	Cardene IV	Hypertension, angina
Nisoldipine	Sular	Hypertension
Olanzapine	Zyprexa	Psychotic disorders
Olanzapine/fluoxetine	Symbyax	Bipolar disorder/depression
Olmesartan	Benicar	Hypertension
Olmesartan/HCTZ	Benicar HCT	Hypertension

Olopatadine (ophthalmic solution)	Patanol	Allergic conjunctivitis
Omega-3 acid ethyl esters	Lovaza	Hypertriglyceridemia
Ondansetron	Zofran	Nausea/vomiting
Oseltamivir	Tamiflu	Influenza A or B
Oxaliplatin	Eloxatin	Colon or rectal cancer (metastatic)
Oxcarbazepine	Trileptal	Partial seizures (children)
Oxycodone	OxyContin	Pain
Oxycodone/acetaminophen	Endocet, Roxicet	Pain
Paclitaxel	Taxol	Various cancers
Palonosetron	Aloxi	Nausea/vomiting
Pantoprazole	Protonix	GERD, erosive esophagitis
Paroxetine (controlled release)	Paxil CR	Depression, OCD, panic disorder, social anxiety, PMDD, PTSD
Phenytoin	Dilantin Kapseals	Seizures
Pimecrolimus	Elidel	Eczema

Pioglitazone	Actos	Diabetes type 2
Piperacillin/tazobactam	Zosyn	Bacterial infections
Polyethylene glycol electrolyte solution	GlycoLax	Bowel cleansing
Potassium chloride	Klor-Con	Potassium replacement
Pramipexole	Mirapex	Parkinson's disease
Pregabalin	Lyrica	Seizures, fibromyalgia, diabetic neuropathy
Progesterone	Prometrium	Amenorrhea, uterine bleeding
Quetiapine	Seroquel	Psychotic disorders
Rabeprazole	Aciphex	GERD, duodenal ulcer, hypersecretory disorders
Raloxifene	Evista	Osteoporosis prevention
Ramelteon	Rozerem	Insomnia
Ramipril	Altace	Hypertension, heart failure
Risedronate	Actonel	Osteoporosis, Paget's disease
Risperidone	Risperdal	Psychotic disorders
Rituximab	Rituxan	Rheumatoid arthritis, non-Hodgkin's lymphoma

Top 200 Drugs (CONTINUED)

Ropinirole	Requip	Parkinson's disease, restless leg syndrome
Rosiglitazone	Avandia	Diabetes type 2
Rosiglitazone/glimepiride	Avandaryl	Diabetes
Rosiglitazone/metformin	Avandamet	Diabetes
Rosuvastatin	Crestor	Hyperlipidemia
Salmeterol (inhalation)	Serevent Diskus	Asthma, COPD, bronchospasm
Sertraline	Zoloft	Depression, social anxiety, OCD, PMDD
Sildenafil	Viagra	Erectile dysfunction
Simvastatin	Zocor	Hyperlipidemia, CHD
Sitagliptin	Januvia	Diabetes
Solifenacin succinate	VESIcare	Overactive bladder
Sumatriptan	Imitrex Oral	Migraine
Tacrolimus	Prograf	Prevent organ transplant rejection
Tadalafil	Cialis	Erectile dysfunction
Tamsulosin	Flomax	BPH

Telmisartan	Micardis	Hypertension
Thyroid	Thyroid	Hypothyroidism
Tobramycin/dexamethasone (ophthalmic suspension)	TobraDex	Ocular infection/inflammation
Tolterodine (long acting)	Detrol LA	Bladder instability
Topiramate	Topamax	Seizures
Tramadol	Ultram, Ultram ER	Pain
Tramadol/acetaminophen	Ultracet	Short-term treatment of pain
Travoprost (ocular)	Travatan	Open-angle glaucoma, ocular hypertension
Triamcinolone (nasal spray)	Nasacort AQ	Allergies
Valacyclovir	Valtrex	Herpes, shingles, cold sores, CMV disease
Valproic acid	Depakote, Depakote ER	Seizures
Valsartan	Diovan	Hypertension, CHF
Valsartan/HCTZ	Diovan HCT	Hypertension
Vancomycin	Vancomycin	Bacterial infections

Top 200 Drugs (continued)

Vardenafil	Levitra	Erectile dysfunction
Varenicline	Chantix	Smoking cessation
Venlafaxine (extended release)	Effexor XR	Depression, social anxiety disorder, panic disorder
Verapamil (sustained release)	Calan SR	Angina, hypertension
Warfarin	Coumadin	Preventive therapy for blood clots
Zaleplon	Sonata	Insomnia
Ziprasidone	Geodon	Schizophrenia, bipolar mania
Zoledronic acid	Zometa	Hypercalcemia related to cancer, osteoporosis, Paget's disease
Zolpidem	Ambien CR, Ambien	Insomnia

The Drug Enforcement Administration (DEA) has the authority to specify which drugs need special controls. These drugs are defined in five categories of controlled substances:

- *Schedule I* drugs have high abuse and addiction potential and have no accepted medical use in the United States. Examples include heroin, LSD, marijuana, mescaline, 3,4-methylenedioxymethamphetamine ("Ecstasy"), psilocin ("mushrooms"), and fentanyl ("China White").
- *Schedule II* drugs have high abuse and addiction potential but do have medical applications. Examples include cocaine, Dilaudid (hydromorphone), Ritalin (methylphenidate), Seconal (secobarbital), MS Contin (morphine), various opiate analgesics, and several types of amphetamines ("diet pills" or "speed").
- *Schedule III* drugs have abuse and addiction potential but not as much as those in Schedule II. Examples include Tylenol #3 (acetaminophen with codeine), Fastin (phentermine), anabolic steroids, and Marinol (THC).
- *Schedule IV* drugs have a low potential for abuse. Examples include Valium (diazepam), Halcion (triazolam), Darvon (propoxyphene), Somnote (chloral hydrate), Ambien (zolpidem), Versed (midazolam), and Talwin.
- *Schedule V* drugs have low abuse potential and have very limited amounts of drugs in each dosage form. Examples are Lomotil (diphenoxylate and atropine) and some cough syrups containing codeine. Some Schedule V products do not even require a prescription (because of FDA regulations), but they must be dispensed by a pharmacist because of DEA rules.

Source: Posey LM. *Complete Review for the Pharmacy Technician,* 2nd edition. Washington, DC: American Pharmacists Association; 2007.

TRADE NAME INDEX

A

Abelcet (amphotericin B, lipid based), 10

Abilify (aripiprazole), 13

Abilify Discmelt (aripiprazole), 13

Abraxane (paclitaxel, protein bound), 136

Abreva (docosanol), 53

Accolate (zafirlukast), 183

Accupril (quinapril), 150

Accuretic (quinapril/HCTZ), 150

Accutane (isotretinoin), 98

Aceta (acetaminophen), 2

Acetadote (acetylcysteine), 2

Aciphex (rabeprazole), 151

Aclovate (alclometasone), 4

Acova (argatroban), 13

Acticin (permethrin), 141

Actigall (ursodiol), 179

Actiq (fentanyl, oral), 74

Activase (alteplase), 6

Activella (estradiol/ norethindrone), 63

Actonel (risedronate), 155

Actoplus Met (metformin/ pioglitazone), 113

Actos (pioglitazone), 143

Actron (ketoprofen), 99

Acular (ketorolac, ocular), 99

Aczone (dapsone), 44

Adalat (nifedipine), 126

Adalat CC (nifedipine), 126

Adderall (dextroamphetamine/ amphetamine), 48

Adderall XR (dextroamphetamine/ amphetamine), 48

Adipex-P (phentermine), 142

Adrucil (fluorouracil, injection), 77

Advair Diskus (fluticasone/ salmeterol), 79

Advicor (lovastatin/niacin), 108

Advil (ibuprofen), 90

AeroBid (flunisolide, inhaled), 76

Aggrenox (aspirin/ dipyridamole), 14

Agrylin (anagrelide), 11

A-Hydrocort (hydrocortisone sodium succinate), 89

Akarpine (pilocarpine, ocular), 142

AKBeta (levobunolol), 103

AK-Chlor (chloramphenicol, ocular), 34

AK-Con (naphazoline), 124

AK-Dex (dexamethasone, ocular), 47

Akineton (biperiden), 20

Akne-mycin (erythromycin, topical), 60

AKPro (dipivefrin), 52

AKTob (tobramycin, ocular), 172

AK-Tracin (bacitracin), 16

Albalon (naphazoline), 124

Aldactone (spironolactone), 162

Aldara (imiquimod), 92

Aldomet (methyldopa), 114

Aldoril (methyldopa/HCTZ), 114

Aldurazyme (laronidase), 101

Alesse (ethinyl estradiol/
levonorgestrel), 67

Aleve (naproxen), 124

Alimta (pemetrexed), 139

Alinia (nitazoxanide), 127

Allegra (fexofenadine), 75

Allegra-D (fexofenadine/
pseudoephedrine), 75

Alomide (lodoxamide), 106

Alora (estradiol, transdermal),
62

Aloxi (palonosetron), 137

Alphagan (brimonidine), 22

Alphagan-P (brimonidine), 22

Alphatrex (betamethasone
diproprionate), 19

Alprazolam Intensol
(alprazolam), 6

Aplenzin (bupropion), 24

Alrex (loteprednol), 108

Altabax (retapamulin), 153

Altace (ramipril), 152

Altocor (lovastatin), 108

Alupent (metaproterenol), 112

Amaryl (glimepiride), 84

Ambien (zolpidem), 184

Ambien CR (zolpidem), 184

AmBisome (amphotericin B,
lipid based), 10

Amen (medroxyprogesterone
acetate), 110

Amerge (naratriptan), 124

A-Methapred
(methylprednisolone sodium
succinate), 115

Amevive (alefacept), 4

Amicar (aminocaproic acid), 7

Amigesic (salsalate), 158

Amikin (amikacin), 7

Amitiza (lubiprostone), 109

Amoxil (amoxicillin), 9

Amphadase (hyaluronidase), 87

Amphocin (amphotericin B
desoxycholate, nonlipid
based), 10

Amphotec (amphotericin B,
lipid based), 10

Anafranil (clomipramine), 39

Anaprox DS (naproxen), 124

Ancef (cefazolin), 29

Ancobon (flucytosine), 75

Androderm (testosterone,
transdermal), 168

Androgel (testosterone,
topical), 168

Angeliq (estradiol/
drospirenone), 62

Angiomax (bivalirudin), 21

Ansaid (flurbiprofen, oral), 78

Antabuse (disulfiram), 52

Antara (fenofibrate), 73

Anthra-Derm (anthralin), 12

Antivert (meclizine), 110

Antrizine (meclizine), 110

Anturane (sulfinpyrazone), 164

Anzemet (dolasetron), 53

Apidra (insulin, glulisine), 93

Apokyn (apomorphine), 12

Apresazide (hydralazine/ HCTZ), 88

Apresoline (hydralazine), 88

Apri (ethinyl estradiol/ desogestrel), 65

Aptivus (tipranavir), 172

Aquachloral Supprettes (chloral hydrate), 34

Aqua-Mephyton (vitamin K [phytonadione]), 182

Aralen (chloroquine phosphate), 35

Aranesp (darbepoetin alfa), 45

Arava (leflunomide), 101

Arcalyst (rilonacept), 155

Aricept (donepezil), 53

Aricept ODT (donepezil), 53

Arimidex (anastrozole), 11

Aristocort (triamcinolone, oral), 177

Aristocort (triamcinolone acetonide), 177

Arixtra (fondaparinux sodium), 80

Armour-Thyroid (thyroid desiccated), 170

Aromasin (exemestane), 72

Arranon (nelarabine), 125

Artane (trihexyphenidyl), 178

Arthrotec (diclofenac/ misoprostol), 49

Asacol (mesalamine), 112

Asendin (amoxapine), 9

Asimia (paroxetine), 138

Asmanex (mometasone furoate), 121

Astelin (azelastine, nasal), 15

Atacand (candesartan), 26

Atarax (hydroxyzine), 90

Ativan (lorazepam), 107

Atridox (doxycycline), 55

Atripla (efavirenz/emtricitabine/ tenofovir disoproxil fumarate), 56

Atrovent (ipratropium), 96

Augmentin (amoxicillin/ clavulanate), 10

Augmentin ES (amoxicillin/ clavulanate), 10

Augmentin XR (amoxicillin/ clavulanate), 10

Avalide (irbesartan/HCTZ), 96

Avandamet (rosiglitazone/ metformin), 157

Avandaryl (rosiglitazone/ glimepiride), 157

Avandia (rosiglitazone), 157

Avapro (irbesartan), 96

Avastin (bevacizumab), 20

Avelox (moxifloxacin), 122

Aventyl (nortriptyline), 130

Aviane (ethinyl estradiol/ levonorgestrel), 67

Avinza (morphine), 121

Avodart (dutasteride), 55

Avonex (interferon beta-1a), 95

Axert (almotriptan), 5

Axid (nizatidine), 129

Axid AR (nizatidine), 129

Aygestin (norethindrone acetate), 129

Azactam (aztreonam), 16

AzaSite (azithromycin, ocular), 16

Azilect (rasagiline), 153

Azmacort (triamcinolone, inhaled), 176

Azopt (brinzolamide), 22

Azor (amlodipine/olmesartan), 9

Azulfidine (sulfasalazine), 163

Azulfidine EN (sulfasalazine), 163

B

Bactrim (trimethoprim/sulfamethoxazole), 178

Bactroban (mupirocin), 122

Balacet (propoxyphene/acetaminophen), 148

Baraclude (entecavir), 58

Barbita (phenobarbital), 142

Beclovent (beclomethasone, inhaled), 17

Beconase (beclomethasone, nasal), 17

Beconase AQ (beclomethasone, nasal), 17

Beepen-VK (penicillin VK), 140

Benadryl (diphenhydramine), 51

Benemid (probenecid), 147

Benicar (olmesartan), 131

Benicar HCT (olmesartan/HCTZ), 131

Bentyl (dicyclomine), 50

Benzac (benzoyl peroxide), 18

BenzaClin (benzoyl peroxide/clindamycin, topical), 18

Benzamycin (erythromycin/benzoyl peroxide), 61

Betachron ER (propranolol), 149

Betagan (levobunolol), 103

Betapace (sotalol), 162

Betapace AF (sotalol), 162

Betaseron (interferon beta-1b), 95

Betatrex (betamethasone valerate), 19

Betaxon (levobetaxolol), 102

Betimol (timolol, ocular), 171

Betoptic (betaxolol, ocular), 19

Betoptic S (betaxolol, ocular), 19

Bexxar (tositumomab/iodine I 131 tositumomab), 175

Biaxin (clarithromycin), 38

Biaxin XL (clarithromycin), 38

Bicillin LA (penicillin G benzathine), 139

BiDil (hydralazine/isosorbide), 88

Biocef (cephalexin), 32

Biothroid (thyroid desiccated), 170

Blocadren (timolol, oral), 171

Boniva (ibandronate), 90
Botox (botulinum toxin type A), 22
Brethine (terbutaline), 167
Brevicon (ethinyl estradiol/ norethindrone), 68
Bronkosol (isoetharine), 97
Brovana (arformoterol), 13
Budeprion SR (bupropion), 24
Bumex (bumetanide), 23
Buprenex (buprenorphine, sublingual), 24
Buproban (bupropion), 24
BuSpar (buspirone), 24
Butisol (butabarbital), 25
Byclomine (dicyclomine), 50
Byetta (exenatide), 72
Bystolic (nebivolol), 124

C

Ca-DTPA (pentetate calcium trisodium), 140
Caduet (amlodopine/ atorvastatin), 8
Calan (verapamil), 181
Calan SR (verapamil), 181
Calcium Chloride (calcium chloride), 26
Calcium Gluconate (calcium gluconate), 26
Campath (alemtuzumab), 4
Campral (acamprosate calcium), 1
Cancidas (caspofungin acetate), 28

Capoten (captopril), 26
Capozide (captopril/HCTZ), 27
Carafate (sucralfate), 163
Cardene (nicardipine), 126
Cardene IV (nicardipine), 126
Cardene SR (nicardipine), 126
Cardizem CD (diltiazem), 51
Cardizem LA (diltiazem), 51
Cardura (doxazosin), 54
Cartrol (carteolol, oral), 28
Casodex (bicalutamide), 20
Cataflam (diclofenac, oral), 49
Catapres (clonidine), 40
Catapres-TTS (clonidine), 40
Cathflo-Activase (alteplase), 6
Ceclor (cefaclor), 28
Cedax (ceftibuten), 31
Cefizox (ceftizoxime sodium), 31
Cefobid (cefoperazone), 30
Ceftin (cefuroxime axetil), 32
Cefzil (cefprozil), 31
Celebrex (celecoxib), 32
Celexa (citalopram), 38
CellCept (mycophenolate mofetil), 122
Cenestin (estrogens A, conjugated, synthetic), 63
Ceptaz (ceftazidime), 31
Cerebyx (fosphenytoin), 81
Cesamet (nabilone), 122
Cetrotide (cetrorelix acetate), 33
Chantix (varenicline), 181
Chibroxin (norfloxacin, ocular), 129

Chloromycetin (chloramphenicol, oral), 34

Chloroptic (chloramphenicol, ocular), 34

Cialis (tadalafil), 165

Ciloxan (ciprofloxacin, ocular), 37

Cimzia (certolizumab pegol), 33

Cinobac (cinoxacin), 37

Cipro (ciprofloxacin), 37

Ciprodex (ciprofloxacin/ dexamethasone, otic), 37

Cipro HC (ciprofloxacin/ hydrocortisone, otic), 38

Cipro XR (ciprofloxacin), 37

Claforan (cefotaxime sodium), 30

Clarinex (desloratadine), 46

Clarinex-D 12 Hour (desloratadine/ pseudoephedrine), 46

Clarinex-D 24 Hour (desloratadine/ pseudoephedrine), 46

Clarinex Redi-tabs (desloratadine), 46

Claritin (loratadine), 107

Claritin-D (loratadine/ pseudoephedrine), 107

Claritin-D 24 Hour (loratadine/ pseudoephedrine), 107

Cleocin (clindamycin), 38

Cleocin(clindamycin,vaginal),39

Cleocin T (clindamycin, topical), 39

Cleviprex (clevidipine butyrate), 38

Climara (estradiol, transdermal), 62

Climara Pro (estradiol/ levonorgestrel, transdermal), 62

Clinda-Derm (clindamycin, topical), 39

Clindesse (clindamycin, vaginal), 39

Clinoril (sulindac), 164

Clolar (clofarabine), 39

Clopra (metoclopramide), 116

Cloxapen (cloxacillin), 41

Clozaril (clozapine), 41

Codeine (codeine sulfate), 41

Cogentin (benztropine), 18

Cognex (tacrine), 165

Colazal (balsalazide), 17

Colchicine (colchicine), 41

Combigan (brimonidine/ timolol), 22

Combipres (clonidine/ chlorthalidone), 40

Combivent (ipratropium/ albuterol), 96

Combivir (lamivudine/ zidovudine), 100

Compazine (prochlorperazine), 147

Comtan (entacapone), 58

Concerta (methylphenidate), 115

Cordarone (amiodarone), 8

Cordarone IV (amiodarone), 8
Coreg (carvedilol), 28
Coreg CR (carvedilol), 28
Corgard (nadolol), 123
Cort-Dome (hydrocortisone, topical), 89
Cortef (hydrocortisone, oral), 89
Cosopt (dorzolamide/timolol), 54
Cotrim (trimethoprim/ sulfamethoxazole), 178
Coumadin (warfarin), 183
Cozaar (losartan), 107
Crestor (rosuvastatin), 157
Crixivan (indinavir), 92
Crolom (cromolyn, ocular), 42
Cryselle (ethinyl estradiol/ norgestrel), 71
Cubicin (daptomycin), 44
Cutivate (fluticasone propionate, topical), 79
Cyclocort (amcinonide), 7
Cycrin (medroxyprogesterone acetate), 110
Cymbalta (duloxetine), 55
Cytomel (liothyronine), Cytotec (misoprostol), 105
Cytovene (ganciclovir), 82
Cytoxan (cyclophosphamide), 43

D

Dacogen (decitabine), 45
Dalalone (dexamethasone sodium phosphate), 48

Dalalone LA (dexamethasone acetate), 47
Dalmane (flurazepam), 77
Dantrium (dantrolene), 44
Darvocet N-50 (propoxyphene napsylate/acetaminophen), 149
Darvocet N-100 (propoxyphene napsylate/acetaminophen), 149
Darvon (propoxyphene), 148
Darvon Compound-65 (propoxyphene/aspirin/ caffeine), 149
Darvon-N (propoxyphene), 148
Daypro (oxaprozin), 134
Daytrana (methylphenidate), 115
Decadron (dexamethasone, oral), 47
Decadron LA (dexamethasone acetate), 47
Decadron Phosphate (dexamethasone sodium phosphate), 48
Declomycin (demeclocycline), 46
Delta-Cortef (prednisolone, oral), 146
Deltasone (prednisone), 146
Demadex (torsemide), 174
Demerol (meperidine), 111
Demulen 1/35 (ethinyl estradiol/ethynodiol), 66
Demulen 1/50 (ethinyl estradiol/ethynodiol), 66

Denavir (penciclovir), 139

Depade (naltrexone), 123

Depakene (valproic acid and derivatives), 180

Depakote (valproic acid and derivatives), 180

Depakote ER (valproic acid and derivatives), 180

DepoDur (morphine sulfate, liposomal), 121

Depoject (methylprednisolone acetate), 115

Depo-Medrol (methylprednisolone acetate), 115

Deponit (nitroglycerin, transdermal), 128

Depopred (methylprednisolone acetate), 115

Depo-Provera (medroxyprogesterone acetate), 110

Depo-SubQ Provera (medroxyprogesterone acetate), 110

Dermacort (hydrocortisone, topical), 89

Desogen (ethinyl estradiol/ desogestrel), 65

DesOwen (desonide), 47

Detrol (tolterodine), 174

Detrol LA (tolterodine), 174

Dexasone (dexamethasone sodium phosphate), 48

Dexedrine (dextroamphetamine sulfate), 48

Dexone (dexamethasone, oral), 47

Diabeta (glyburide), 84

Diabinese (chlorpropamide), 35

Didronel (etidronate), 71

Differin (adapalene), 3

Diflucan (fluconazole), 75

Diflucan IV (fluconazole), 75

Digitek (digoxin), 50

Dilacor XR (diltiazem), 51

Dilantin (phenytoin), 142

Diovan (valsartan), 180

Diovan HCT (valsartan/HCTZ), 180

Dipentum (olsalazine), 132

Diprosone (betamethasone diproprionate), 19

Disalcid (salsalate), 158

Di-Spaz (dicyclomine), 50

Ditropan (oxybutynin), 135

Ditropan XL (oxybutynin), 135

Diuril (chlorothiazide), 35

Divigel (estradiol, gel), 61

Dobutrex (dobutamine), 52

Dolobid (diflunisal), 50

Doral (quazepam), 150

Doribax (doripenem), 53

Dostinex (cabergoline), 25

Dovonex (calcipotriene), 25

Doxy (doxycycline), 54

Doxychel (doxycycline), 54

Dramanate (dimenhydrinate), 51

Drithocreme (anthralin), 12

Duac (benzoyl peroxide/
  clindamycin, topical), 18
Duetact (pioglitazone/
  glimepiride), 143
Duragesic (fentanyl,
  transdermal), 74
Duramorph (morphine), 121
Durezol (difluprednate, ocular),
  50
Duricef (cefadroxil), 29
Dycill (dicloxacillin), 49
Dymelor (acetohexamide), 2
Dynabac (dirithromycin), 52
Dynacin (minocycline), 119
DynaCirc (isradipine), 98
DynaCirc CR (isradipine), 98
Dynapen (dicloxacillin), 49
Dyrenium (triamterene), 177

E
E-Base (erythromycin, base),
  59
Econopred (prednisolone,
  ocular), 145
Edecrin (ethacrynic acid), 65
EES (erythromycin
  ethylsuccinate), 60
Effexor (venlafaxine), 181
Effexor XR (venlafaxine), 181
Efudex (fluorouracil, topical),
  77
Elaprase (idursulfase), 91
Elavil (amitriptyline), 8
Eldepryl (selegiline), 159
Elestat (epinastine, ocular), 58

Elidel (pimecrolimus), 143
Elimite (permethrin), 141
Elitek (rasburicase), 153
Elocon (mometasone, topical),
  120
Eloxatin (oxaliplatin), 134
Emadine (emedastine), 57
Emend (aprepitant), 12
Emend (fosaprepitant
  dimeglumine), 80
Emgel (erythromycin, topical),
  60
Empirin (aspirin), 13
Emsam (selegiline), 159
Emtriva (emtricitabine), 57
E-Mycin (erythromycin, base),
  59
Enablex (darifenacin
  hydrobromide), 45
Enbrel (etanercept), 64
Endocet (oxycodone/
  acetaminophen), 135
Enjuvia (estrogens B,
  conjugated, synthetic), 64
Enpresse (ethinyl estradiol/
  levonorgestrel), 68
Entereg (alvimopan), 6
Entocort EC (budesonide), 23
Eovist (gadoxetate disodium),
  82
Epifrin (epinephrine), 58
Epitol (carbamazepine), 27
Epivir (lamivudine [3TC]), 100
Epivir-HBV (lamivudine [3TC]),
  100

Epogen (epoetin alfa), 59

Epzicom (abacavir/lamivudine), 1

Equetro (carbamazepine), 27

Eraxis (anidulafungin), 12

Erbitux (cetuximab), 33

Ergomar (ergotamine tartrate), 59

Ertaczo (sertaconazole, topical), 160

Eryc (erythromycin, base), 59

Erygel (erythromycin, topical), 60

EryPed (erythromycin ethylsuccinate), 60

Ery-Tab (erythromycin, base), 59

Erythrocin (erythromycin lactobionate), 60

Erythrocin (erythromycin stearate), 60

Esidrix (hydrochlorothiazide), 88

Eskalith (lithium), 106

Eskalith CR (lithium), 106

Estinyl (ethinyl estradiol), 65

Estraderm (estradiol, transdermal), 62

Estrasorb (estradiol, 17-beta, topical emulsion), 62

Estratab (estrogens, esterified), 63

EstroGel (estradiol, gel), 61

Estrostep (ethinyl estradiol/ norethindrone), 70

Estrostep Fe (ethinyl estradiol/ norethindrone), 70

Ethmozine (moricizine), 121

Etrafon (perphenazine/ amitriptyline), 141

Eulexin (flutamide), 78

Eurax (crotamiton), 42

Evamist (estradiol, spray), 62

Evista (raloxifene), 151

Evoxac (cevimeline), 33

Exelon (rivastigmine), 156

Exelon (rivastigmine, transdermal), 156

Exforge (amlodipine/valsartan), 9

Exjade (deferasirox), 45

Exubera (insulin, human [rDNA]), 93

F

Fabrazyme (agalsidase beta), 3

Factive (gemifloxacin), 83

Famvir (famciclovir), 73

Fareston (toremifene), 174

Faslodex (fulvestrant), 81

Fastin (phentermine), 142

Feldene (piroxicam), 144

Femara (letrozole), 102

FemPatch (estradiol, transdermal), 62

Femring (estradiol, vaginal ring), 62

Fentora (fentanyl, buccal), 74

5-FU (fluorouracil, injection), 77

Flagyl (metronidazole), 117

Flagyl IV (metronidazole), 117

Flarex (fluorometholone), 76

Flector (diclofenac epolamine, transdermal), 49

Flexeril (cyclobenzaprine), 43

Flomax (tamsulosin), 165

Flonase (fluticasone, nasal), 78

Flo-Pred (prednisolone, oral), 146

Flovent (fluticasone, inhaled), 78

Floxin (ofloxacin), 130

Floxin Otic (ofloxacin, otic), 131

Flumadine (rimantadine), 155

FluMist (influenza virus vaccine, live, intranasal), 93

Fluonex (fluocinonide), 76

Fluonid (fluocinolone), 76

Fluor-Op (fluorometholone), 76

Fluoroplex (fluorouracil, topical), 77

Flurosyn (fluocinolone), 76

Flutex (triamcinolone acetonide), 177

FML (fluorometholone), 76

Focalin (dexmethylphenidate), 48

Focalin XR (dexmethylphenidate), 48

Foltx (folic acid/ cyanocobalamin/pyridoxine), 79

Foradil (formoterol), 80

Fortamet (metformin), 113

Fortaz (ceftazidime), 31

Forteo (teriparatide), 168

Fortical (calcitonin-salmon [rDNA origin]), 26

Fosamax (alendronate), 4

Fosamax Plus D (alendronate/ cholecalciferol), 4

Foscavir (foscarnet), 80

Fosrenol (lanthanum carbonate), 101

Fragmin (dalteparin sodium), 44

Frova (frovatriptan), 81

Fulvicin (griseofulvin microsize), 85

Fulvicin P/G (griseofulvin ultramicrosize), 85

Fungizone (amphotericin B), 10

Furadantin (nitrofurantoin), 127

Fusilev (levoleucovorin), 104

Fuzeon (enfuvirtide), 57

G

Gabitril (tiagabine), 170

Garamycin (gentamicin), 83

Garamycin (gentamicin, injection), 84

Gardasil (human papillomavirus vaccine), 87

Gastrocrom (cromolyn, oral), 42

Genoptic (gentamicin), 83

Genora 0.5/35 (ethinyl estradiol/norethindrone), 68

Genora 1/35 (ethinyl estradiol/ norethindrone), 68

Genora 1/50 (mestranol/
  norethindrone), 112
Gentak (gentamicin), 83
Gen-Xene (clorazepate), 40
Geocillin (carbenicillin), 27
Geodon (ziprasidone), 184
Glaucon (epinephrine), 58
Gleevec (imatinib), 91
Glucophage (metformin), 113
Glucophage XR (metformin), 113
Glucotrol (glipizide), 84
Glucotrol XL (glipizide), 84
Glucovance (glyburide/
  metformin), 84
Glumetza (metformin), 113
GlycoLax (polyethylene glycol),
  144
Glynase (glyburide), 84
Glyset (miglitol), 118
Grifulvin (griseofulvin
  microsize), 85
Grisactin (griseofulvin
  ultramicrosize), 85
Gris-PEG (griseofulvin
  ultramicrosize), 85
Guaifenex PSE (guaifenesin/
  pseudoephedrine), 85
G-well (lindane), 105

H
Halcion (triazolam), 177
Haldol (haloperidol), 86
Halfan (halofantrine), 86
Halog (halcinonide), 86
Halog-E (halcinonide), 86

Halotex (haloprogin), 86
Heparin (heparin), 87
Hepsera (adefovir dipivoxil), 3
Herplex (idoxuridine), 91
Hespan (hetastarch), 87
Hexadrol (dexamethasone,
  oral), 47
Humalog (insulin, lispro), 94
Humalog 75/25 (insulin, lispro
  protamine suspension and
  insulin lispro), 94
Humatin (paromomycin), 138
Humira (adalimumab), 3
Humulin 50/50 (insulin,
  isophane suspension and
  insulin regular), 94
Humulin L (insulin, zinc
  suspension), 94
Humulin N (insulin, isophane
  suspension), 94
Humulin R (insulin, regular), 94
Humulin 70/30 (insulin,
  isophane suspension and
  insulin regular), 94
Humulin U (insulin, zinc
  suspension, extended), 95
Hycort (hydrocortisone,
  topical), 89
Hydase (hyaluronidase), 87
Hydrate (dimenhydrinate), 51
Hydrocortone Acetate
  (hydrocortisone acetate), 89
HydroDIURIL
  (hydrochlorothiazide), 88

Hygroton (chlorthalidone), 35
Hylorel (guanadrel), 85
Hyrexin-50 (diphenhydramine), 51
Hyzaar (losartan/HCTZ), 108

I

Ilosone (erythromycin estolate), 60
Ilotycin (erythromycin, ocular), 60
Imdur (isosorbide mononitrate), 97
Imitrex (sumatriptan), 164
Implanon (etonogestrel), 72
Increlex (mecasermin [rDNA]), 109
Inderal (propranolol), 149
Inderal LA (propranolol), 149
Inderide (propranolol/HCTZ), 149
Inderide LA (propranolol/HCTZ), 149
Indocin (indomethacin), 92
Indocin ER (indomethacin), 92
Indocin SR (indomethacin), 92
Infumorph (morphine), 121
Innohep (tinzaparin), 172
Innopran XL (propranolol), 149
Inspra (eplerenone), 58
Intal (cromolyn, inhaled), 42
Intelence (etravirine), 72
Intron-A (interferon alfa-2b), 95
Intropin (dopamine), 53

Invanz (ertapenem), 59
Invega (paliperidone), 136
Invirase (saquinavir), 159
Ionamin (phentermine), 142
Iopidine (apraclonidine), 12
IPlex (mecasermin rinfabate), 109
Iressa (gefitinib), 83
Isentress (raltegravir potassium), 152
Ismelin (guanethidine), 86
Ismo (isosorbide mononitrate), 97
Isoptin (verapamil), 181
Isoptin SR (verapamil), 181
Isopto Atropine (atropine), 15
Isopto Carpine (pilocarpine, ocular), 142
Isordil (isosorbide dinitrate), 97
Istalol (timolol, ocular), 171
Isuprel (isoproterenol), 97
Ixempra (ixabepilone), 98

J

Janumet (sitagliptin/metformin), 162
Januvia (sitagliptin), 161
Jenest-28 (ethinyl estradiol/norethindrone), 69

K

Kadian (morphine), 121
Kaletra (lopinavir/ritonavir), 107
Kantrex (kanamycin), 98

Kaon-Cl (potassium chloride), 144

Kariva (ethinyl estradiol/ desogestrel), 65

K-Dur (potassium chloride), 144

Keflex (cephalexin), 32

Keftab (cephalexin hydrochloride), 32

Kefzol (cefazolin), 29

Kemadrin (procyclidine), 147

Kenacort (triamcinolone, oral), 177

Kenalog (triamcinolone acetonide), 177

Kepivance (palifermin), 136

Keppra (levetiracetam), 102

Keppra IV (levetiracetam), 102

Kerlone (betaxolol, oral), 19

Ketek (telithromycin), 166

Kineret (anakinra), 11

Klonopin (clonazepam), 39

Klor-Con (potassium chloride), 144

Klorvess (potassium chloride), 144

Klotrix (potassium chloride), 144

K-Lyte (potassium chloride), 144

Kuvan (sapropterin), 158

Kwell (lindane), 105

Kytril (granisetron), 85

L

Lamictal (lamotrigine), 100

Lamisil (terbinafine), 167

Laniazid (isoniazid), 97

Lanoxicaps (digoxin), 50

Lanoxin (digoxin), 50

Lantus (insulin, glargine), 93

Lariam (mefloquine), 110

Lasix (furosemide), 81

Lescol (fluvastatin), 79

Lescol XL (fluvastatin), 79

Lessina (ethinyl estradiol/ levonorgestrel), 67

Letairis (ambrisentan), 7

Levaquin (levofloxacin), 103

Levatol (penbutolol), 139

Levemir (insulin, detemir), 93

Levitra (vardenafil), 180

Levlen (ethinyl estradiol/ levonorgestrel), 67

Levlite (ethinyl estradiol/ levonorgestrel), 67

Levora 0.15/30 (ethinyl estradiol/levonorgestrel), 67

Levo-T (levothyroxine), 104

Levothroid (levothyroxine), 104

Levoxyl (levothyroxine), 104

Levulan Kerastick (aminolevulinic acid), 7

Lexapro (escitalopram), 61

Lexiscan (regadenoson), 153

Lexiva (fosamprenavir), 80

Lialda (mesalamine), 112

Libritabs (chlordiazepoxide), 34

Librium (chlordiazepoxide), 34

Lidex (fluocinonide), 76

Lidoderm (lidocaine), 106

Limbitrol DS (chlordiazepoxide/
amitriptyline), 34
Lioresal (baclofen), 16
Lioresal Intrathecal (baclofen),
16
Lipitor (atorvastatin), 15
Lipofen (fenofibrate), 73
Lithobid (lithium), 106
Lithotabs (lithium), 106
Livostin (levocabastine), 103
Lodine (etodolac), 71
Lodine XL (etodolac), 71
Loestrin 1.5/30 (ethinyl
estradiol/norethindrone), 69
Loestrin 1/20 (ethinyl estradiol/
norethindrone), 69
Loestrin Fe 1/20 (ethinyl
estradiol/norethindrone), 69
Loniten (minoxidil), 119
Lo/Ovral (ethinyl estradiol/
norgestrel), 71
Lopid (gemfibrozil), 83
Lopressor (metoprolol), 116
Lopressor HCT (metoprolol/
HCTZ), 117
Loprox (ciclopirox), 36
Lotemax (loteprednol), 108
Lotensin (benazepril), 17
Lotensin HCT (benazepril/
HCTZ), 18
Lotrel (amlodipine/benazepril),
9
Lotrimin (clotrimazole, topical),
41
Lotronex (alosetron), 6

Lovaza (omega-3 acid ethyl
esters), 132
Lovenox (enoxaparin sodium),
58
Low-Ogestrel (ethinyl estradiol/
norgestrel), 71
Loxitane (loxapine), 108
Loxitane C (loxapine), 108
Lozol (indapamide), 92
Lucentis (ranibizumab), 152
Ludiomil (maprotiline), 109
Lumigan (bimatoprost), 20
Lunesta (eszopiclone), 64
Luvox (fluvoxamine), 79
Luvox CR (fluvoxamine), 79
Lybrel (ethinyl estradiol/
levonorgestrel), 67
Lyrica (pregabalin), 146

M

Macrobid (nitrofurantoin), 127
Macrodantin (nitrofurantoin),
127
Macugen (pegaptanib sodium),
138
Magnesium Sulfate
(magnesium sulfate), 109
Malarone (atovaquone/
proguanil), 15
Malarone-Pediatric
(atovaquone/proguanil), 15
Mandol (cefamandole), 29
Marinol (dronabinol), 55
Marplan (isocarboxazid), 96
Mavik (trandolapril), 175

Maxair (pirbuterol), 144
Maxalt (rizatriptan), 157
Maxalt-MLT (rizatriptan), 157
Maxaquin (lomefloxacin), 106
Maxidex (dexamethasone, ocular), 47
Maxipime (cefepime), 29
Maxivate (betamethasone diproprionate), 19
Maxolon (metoclopramide), 116
Medihaler (isoproterenol), 97
Medrol (methylprednisolone), 115
Mefoxin (cefoxitin sodium), 30
Megace (megestrol acetate), 111
Megace ES (megestrol acetate), 111
Mellaril (thioridazine), 169
Mellaril-S (thioridazine), 169
Menest (estrogens, esterified), 63
Menostar (estradiol, transdermal), 62
Mentax (butenafine), 25
Mephyton (vitamin K [phytonadione]), 182
Meridia (sibutramine), 160
Merrem IV (meropenem), 111
Metadate (methylphenidate), 115
Metadate CD (methylphenidate), 115
Metaglip (metformin/glipizide), 113

Methylin (methylphenidate), 115
Meticorten (prednisone), 146
MetroGel (metronidazole, topical), 117
MetroGel-Vaginal (metronidazole, vaginal), 117
MetroLotion (metronidazole, topical), 117
Mevacor (lovastatin), 108
Mexitil (mexiletine), 117
Mezlin (mezlocillin), 117
Miacalcin (calcitonin), 25
Micardis (telmisartan), 166
Microgestin Fe 1/20 (ethinyl estradiol/norethindrone), 69
Microgestin 1.5/30 (ethinyl estradiol/norethindrone), 69
Micro-K (potassium chloride), 144
Micronase (glyburide), 84
Micronor (norethindrone), 129
Microsulfon (sulfadiazine), 163
Midamor (amiloride), 7
Mifeprex (mifepristone), 118
Migranal (dihydroergotamine), 51
Minipress (prazosin), 145
Minitran (nitroglycerin, transdermal), 128
Minizide (prazosin/polythiazide), 145
Minocin (minocycline), 119
MiraLax (polyethylene glycol), 144

Mirapex (pramipexole), 145

Mircera (methoxy polyethylene glycol epoetin beta), 114

Mircette (ethinyl estradiol/ desogestrel), 65

Mitran (chlordiazepoxide), 34

Moban (molindone), 120

Mobic (meloxicam), 111

Modicon (ethinyl estradiol/ norethindrone), 68

Monistat-Derm (miconazole), 118

Monistat-3 (miconazole), 118

Monocid (cefonicid), 30

Monoket (isosorbide mononitrate), 97

Monopril (fosinopril), 81

Motrin (ibuprofen), 90

MS Contin (morphine), 121

Mucomyst (acetylcysteine), 2

Multihance (gadobenate dimeglumine), 82

Myambutol (ethambutol), 65

Mycamine (micafungin sodium), 118

Mycelex (clotrimazole, oral), 40

Mycelex (clotrimazole, topical), 41

Mycobutin (rifabutin), 154

Mycostatin (nystatin, oral), 130

Mykrox (metolazone), 116

Mylotarg (gemtuzumab ozogamicin), 83

Myobloc (botulinum toxin type B), 22

Myozyme (alglucosidase alfa), 5

Mysoline (primidone), 146

N

Naftin (naftifine), 123

Naglazyme (galsulfase), 82

Nalfon (fenoprofen), 74

Nallpen (nafcillin), 123

Namenda (memantine), 111

Naprelan (naproxen), 124

Narcan (naloxone), 123

Nardil (phenelzine), 141

Nasacort (triamcinolone, nasal), 176

Nasacort AQ (triamcinolone, nasal), 176

Nasalide (flunisolide, nasal), 76

Nasarel (flunisolide, nasal), 76

Nascobal (cyanocobalamin), 42

Nasonex (mometasone, nasal), 120

Natrecor (nesiritide citrate), 125

Nature-Throid (thyroid desiccated), 170

Navane (thiothixene), 170

Navelbine (vinorelbine), 182

Nebcin (tobramycin sulfate),173

NebuPent (pentamidine isethionate), 140

Necon 0.5/35 (ethinyl estradiol/norethindrone), 68

Necon 1/35 (ethinyl estradiol/ norethindrone), 68

Necon 1/50 (mestranol/ norethindrone), 112

Necon 7/7/7 (ethinyl estradiol/ norethindrone), 70

Necon 10/11 (ethinyl estradiol/ norethindrone), 69

Nelova 0.5/35E (ethinyl estradiol/norethindrone), 68

Nelova 1/35E (ethinyl estradiol/ norethindrone), 68

Nelova 1/50M (mestranol/ norethindrone), 112

Nelova 10/11 (ethinyl estradiol/ norethindrone), 69

Nembutal (pentobarbital), 141

Neoral (cyclosporine), 43

Neurontin (gabapentin), 81

Nevanac (nepafenac), 125

Nexavar (sorafenib tosylate), 162

Nexium (esomeprazole), 61

Niaspan (niacin [nicotinic acid]), 126

Nilandron (nilutamide), 127

Nilstat (nystatin, oral), 130

Nimotop (nimodipine), 127

Nitro-Bid (nitroglycerin, topical), 128

Nitro-Bid IV (nitroglycerin, injection), 127

Nitro-Dur (nitroglycerin, transdermal), 128

Nitrogard (nitroglycerin, transmucosal-buccal), 128

Nitroglyn (nitroglycerin, sustained release), 128

Nitrol (nitroglycerin, topical), 128

Nitrolingual (nitroglycerin, sublingual), 128

Nitrong (nitroglycerin, sustained release), 128

NitroQuick (nitroglycerin, sublingual), 128

Nitrostat (nitroglycerin, sublingual), 128

Nitrotab (nitroglycerin, sublingual), 128

Nitro-Time (nitroglycerin, sustained release), 128

Nix (permethrin), 141

Nizoral (ketoconazole), 98

Nolvadex (tamoxifen), 156

Norcuron (vecuronium), 181

Nordette (ethinyl estradiol/ levonorgestrel), 67

Norethin 1/35E (ethinyl estradiol/norethindrone), 68

Norethin 1/50M (mestranol/ norethindrone), 112

Norflex (orphenadrine), 133

Norinyl 1+35 (ethinyl estradiol/ norethindrone), 68

Norinyl 1+50 (mestranol/ norethindrone), 112

Noritate (metronidazole, topical), 117

Normodyne (labetalol), 99

Noroxin (norfloxacin, oral), 129

Norpace (disopyramide), 52

Norpace CR (disopyramide), 52

Norpramin (desipramine), 46

Nor-QD (norethindrone), 129

Nortrel 1/35 (ethinyl estradiol/
    norethindrone), 68
Nortrel 0.5/35 (ethinyl
    estradiol/norethindrone), 68
Norvasc (amlodipine), 8
Norvir (ritonavir), 156
Novolin N (insulin, isophane
    suspension), 94
Novolin R (insulin, regular), 94
Novolin 70/30 (insulin,
    isophane suspension and
    insulin regular), 94
NovoLog (insulin, aspart), 93
Noxafil (posaconazole), 144
Nuprin (ibuprofen), 90
NutreStore (L-glutamine), 104
NuvaRing (ethinyl estradiol/
    etonogestrel), 66
Nuvigil (armodafinil), 13
Nydrazid (isoniazid), 97
Nystatin (nystatin, vaginal), 130

O

Octamide (metoclopramide),
    116
Ocuchlor (chloramphenicol,
    ocular), 34
Ocufen (flurbiprofen, ocular),
    78
Ocuflox (ofloxacin, ocular), 130
Ocupress (carteolol, ocular), 28
Ogen (estropipate), 64
Ogestrel (ethinyl estradiol/
    norgestrel), 71
Olux-E (clobetasol), 39

Omnaris (ciclesonide), 36
Omnicef (cefdinir), 29
Omnipen (ampicillin), 11
Opana (oxymorphone), 136
Opana ER (oxymorphone), 136
OptiPranolol (metipranolol), 116
Optivar (azelastine, ocular), 16
Oracea (doxycycline), 55
Oralet (fentanyl, oral), 74
Oramorph SR (morphine), 121
Orap (pimozide), 143
Orapred ODT (prednisolone,
    oral), 146
Orencia (abatacept), 1
Oretic (hydrochlorothiazide), 88
Orgaran (danaparoid sodium),
    44
Orinase (tolbutamide), 173
Ortho-Cept (ethinyl estradiol/
    desogestrel), 65
Ortho-Cyclen (ethinyl estradiol/
    norgestimate), 70
Ortho-Est (estropipate), 64
Ortho Evra (ethinyl estradiol/
    norelgestromin), 68
Ortho-Novum 1/35 (ethinyl
    estradiol/norethindrone), 68
Ortho-Novum 1/50 (mestranol/
    norethindrone), 112
Ortho-Novum 10/11 (ethinyl
    estradiol/norethindrone), 69
Ortho-Novum 7/7/7 (ethinyl
    estradiol/norethindrone), 70
Ortho-Tri-Cyclen (ethinyl
    estradiol/norgestimate), 70

Orudis (ketoprofen), 99

Orudis KT (ketoprofen), 99

Oruvail (ketoprofen), 99

Ovcon 35 (ethinyl estradiol/
norethindrone), 69

Ovcon 50 (ethinyl estradiol/
norethindrone), 68

Ovral (ethinyl estradiol/
norgestrel), 71

Ovrette (norgestrel), 129

Oxacillin (oxacillin), 134

OxyContin (oxycodone), 135

OxyFast (oxycodone), 135

OxyIR (oxycodone), 135

Oxytrol (oxybutynin,
transdermal), 135

P

Pacerone (amiodarone), 8

Pamelor (nortriptyline), 130

Panasol-S (prednisone), 146

PanOxyl (benzoyl peroxide), 18

Panretin (alitretinoin), 5

Paraflex (chlorzoxazone), 36

Parafon Forte DSC
(chlorzoxazone), 36

Parcopa (levodopa/carbidopa),
103

Paredrine
(hydroxyamphetamine), 89

Parlodel (bromocriptine), 23

Parnate (tranylcypromine), 175

Patanase (olopatadine, nasal),
132

Patanol (olopatadine), 132

Pathocil (dicloxacillin), 49

Pavabid (papaverine), 137

Pavacot (papaverine), 137

Pavulon (pancuronium), 137

Paxil (paroxetine), 138

Paxil CR (paroxetine), 138

PCE (erythromycin, base), 59

Pegasys (peginterferon alfa-
2a), 138

Peg-Intron (peginterferon alfa-
2b), 138

Penetrex (enoxacin), 58

Penicillin G Potassium
(penicillin G, aqueous), 139

Penlac (ciclopirox), 36

Pentam 300 (pentamidine
isethionate), 140

Pentasa (mesalamine), 112

Pentothal (thiopental), 169

Pentoxil (pentoxifylline), 141

Pen-Vee K (penicillin VK), 140

Pepcid (famotidine), 73

Pepcid AC (famotidine), 73

Pepcid RPD (famotidine), 73

Percocet (oxycodone/
acetaminophen), 135

Percolone (oxycodone), 135

Perforomist (formoterol
fumarate), 80

Periactin (cyproheptadine), 44

Permapen (penicillin G
benzathine), 139

Permitil (fluphenazine), 77

Persa-Gel (benzoyl peroxide),
18

Persantine (dipyridamole), 52

Pfizerpen (penicillin G, aqueous), 139

Phenergan (promethazine), 148

Phyllocontin (aminophylline), 7

Pilocar (pilocarpine, ocular), 142

Pilostat (pilocarpine, ocular), 142

Pipracil (piperacillin), 143

Pitocin (oxytocin), 136

Plan B (levonorgestrel), 104

Plaquenil (hydroxychloroquine), 90

Platinol-AQ (cisplatin), 38

Plavix (clopidogrel), 40

Plendil (felodipine), 73

Pletal (cilostazol), 36

Ponstel (mefenamic acid), 110

Portia (ethinyl estradiol/ levonorgestrel), 67

PrandiMet (repaglinide/ metformin), 153

Prandin (repaglinide), 153

Pravachol (pravastatin), 145

Precose (acarbose), 1

Pred Forte (prednisolone, ocular), 145

Pred Mild (prednisolone, ocular), 145

Prednicen-M (prednisone), 146

Prelone (prednisolone, oral), 146

Premarin (estrogens, conjugated), 63

Premarin IV (estrogens, conjugated), 63

Premphase (estrogens/ medroxyprogesterone), 64

Prempro (estrogens/ medroxyprogesterone), 64

Prevacid (lansoprazole), 100

Prevacid/NapraPAC (lansoprazole/naproxen), 101

Preven (ethinyl estradiol/ levonorgestrel), 66

Prezista (darunavir), 45

Prialt (ziconotide), 183

Priftin (rifapentine), 154

Prilosec (omeprazole), 132

Primaquine (primaquine), 146

Primaxin (imipenem/cilastatin), 91

Principen (ampicillin), 11

Prinivil (lisinopril), 106

Prinzide (lisinopril/HCTZ), 106

Pristiq (desvenlafaxine), 47

Probalan (probenecid), 147

Pro-Banthine (propantheline), 148

Procanbid (procainamide), 147

Procardia (nifedipine), 126

Procardia XL (nifedipine), 126

Procrit (epoetin alfa), 59

Profenal (suprofen), 164

Prograf (tacrolimus), 165

Prolixin (fluphenazine), 77

Promethegan (promethazine), 148

Prometrium (progesterone), 147

Pronestyl (procainamide), 147

Propecia (finasteride), 75

Propine (dipivefrin), 52

Propylthiouracil (propylthiouracil), 149

Proquin XR (ciprofloxacin), 37

Proscar (finasteride), 75

ProSom (estazolam), 61

Protonix (pantoprazole), 137

Proventil (albuterol), Proventil HFA (albuterol), 3

Provera (medroxyprogesterone acetate), 110

Provigil (modafinil), 120

Prozac (fluoxetine), 77

Prozac Weekly (fluoxetine), 77

Pulmicort (budesonide, inhaled), 23

Pylera (bismuth subcitrate potassium/metronidazole/tetracycline), 20

Pyrazinamide (pyrazinamide), 150

Q

Quinaglute (quinidine gluconate), 151

Quinalan (quinidine gluconate), 151

Quinaretic (quinapril/HCTZ), 150

Quinidex Extentabs (quinidine sulfate), 151

Quinine (quinine sulfate), 151

Quinora (quinidine sulfate), 151

QVAR (beclomethasone, inhaled), 17

R

Ranexa (ranolazine), 152

Rapamune (sirolimus), 161

Raptiva (efalizumab), 56

Razadyne (galantamine), 82

Razadyne ER (galantamine), 82

Rebetrol (ribavirin, oral), 154

Rebif (interferon beta-1a), 95

Reclast (zoledronic acid), 184

Reclomide (metoclopramide), 116

Refludan (lepirudin), 102

Reglan (metoclopramide), 116

Regranex (becaplermin), 17

Relafen (nabumetone), 123

Relenza (zanamivir), 183

Relistor (methylnaltrexone), 114

Relpax (eletriptan), 56

Remeron (mirtazapine), 119

Remicade (infliximab), 92

Remodulin (treprostinil sodium), 176

Remular (chlorzoxazone), 36

Renagel (sevelamer hydrochloride), 160

Renvela (sevelamer carbonate), 160

Requip (ropinirole), 157

Requip XL (ropinirole), 157

Rescriptor (delavirdine), 46

Rescula (unoprostone isopropyl), 179

Restasis (cyclosporine, ocular), 43

Restoril (temazepam), 166

Retavase (reteplase), 154

Retin-A (tretinoin, topical), 176

Retin-A Micro (tretinoin, topical), 176

Retisert (fluocinolone acetonide), 76

Retrovir (zidovudine), 183

Revatio (sildenafil citrate), 161

ReVia (naltrexone), 123

Revlimid (lenalidomide), 102

Reyataz (atazanavir sulfate), 14

Rheumatrex (methotrexate), 113

Rhinocort (budesonide, nasal), 23

Rhinocort Aqua (budesonide, nasal), 23

Ridaura (auranofin), 15

Rifadin (rifampin), 154

Rilutek (riluzole), 155

Rimactane (rifampin), 154

Risperdal (risperidone), 156

Risperdal Consta (risperidone), 156

Ritalin (methylphenidate), 115

Ritalin LA (methylphenidate), 115

Rituxan (rituximab), 156

Robaxin (methocarbamol), 113

Rocephin (ceftriaxone sodium), 31

Roferon-A (interferon alfa-2a), 95

RotaTeq (rotavirus vaccine, live), 158

Rowasa Rectal (mesalamine), 112

Roxanol (morphine), 121

Roxicet (oxycodone/ acetaminophen), 135

Roxicet 5/500 (oxycodone/ acetaminophen), 135

Roxicodone (oxycodone), 135

Roxilox (oxycodone/ acetaminophen), 135

Rozerem (ramelteon), 152

Rythmol (propafenone), 148

S

Salagen (pilocarpine, oral), 142

Salsitab (salsalate), 158

Sanctura (trospium), 179

Sanctura XR (trospium), 179

Sandimmune (cyclosporine), 43

Sandostatin (octreotide), 130

Sandostatin LAR Depot (octreotide), 130

SangCya (cyclosporine), 43

Sansert (methysergide), 116

Sarafem (fluoxetine), 77

Seasonale (ethinyl estradiol/ levonorgestrel), 67

Seasonique (ethinyl estradiol/ levonorgestrel), 67

Seconal (secobarbital), 159

SecreFlo (secretin), 159

Sectral (acebutolol), 1

Selzentry (maraviroc), 109

Sensipar (cinacalcet), 36

Septra (trimethoprim/
  sulfamethoxazole), 178

Serax (oxazepam), 134

Serentil (mesoridazine), 112

Serevent (salmeterol), 158

Serevent Diskus (salmeterol),
  158

Seromycin (cycloserine), 43

Seroquel (quetiapine), 150

Seroquel XR (quetiapine), 150

Serzone (nefazodone), 125

Simcor(simvastatin/niacin),161

Sinemet (levodopa/carbidopa),
  103

Sinemet CR (levodopa/
  carbidopa), 103

Sinequan (doxepin, oral), 54

Singulair (montelukast), 121

Skelaxin (metaxalone), 112

Skelid (tiludronate), 171

Slo-Phyllin (theophylline), 169

Solage(mequinol/tretinoin), 111

Solfoton (phenobarbital), 142

Soliris (eculizumab), 56

Solodyn (minocycline), 119

Soltamox (tamoxifen), 165

Solu-Cortef (hydrocortisone
  sodium succinate), 89

Solu-Medrol
  (methylprednisolone sodium
  succinate), 115

Soma (carisoprodol), 27

Somatuline Depot (lanreotide),
  100

Somavert (pegvisomant), 139

Sonata (zaleplon), 183

Sorbitrate (isosorbide
  dinitrate), 97

Soriatane (acitretin), 2

Sotradecol (sodium tetradecyl
  sulfate), 162

Spectazole (econazole), 56

Spectracef (cefditoren pivoxil),
  29

Spiriva (tiotropium), 172

Sporanox (itraconazole), 98

Sprintec (ethinyl estradiol/
  norgestimate), 70

Sprycel (dasatinib), 45

Stalevo (carbidopa/levodopa/
  entacapone), 27

Starlix (nateglinide), 124

Stelazine (trifluoperazine), 177

Strattera (atomoxetine), 14

Streptase (streptokinase), 163

Striant (testosterone, buccal),
  168

Sublimaze (fentanyl, injection),
  74

Suboxone (buprenorphine/
  naloxone, sublingual), 24

Subutex (buprenorphine,
  sublingual), 24

Sucraid (sacrosidase), 158

Sular (nisoldipine), 127

Sumycin (tetracycline), 168

Suprax (cefixime), 30
Surmontil (trimipramine), 178
Sustiva (efavirenz), 56
Sutent (sunitinib malate), 164
Symbyax (olanzapine/
 fluoxetine), 131
Symlin (pramlintide acetate),
 145
Symmetrel (amantadine), 6
Synalar (fluocinolone), 76
Synera (lidocaine/tetracaine),
 105
Synthroid (levothyroxine), 104
Syntocinon (oxytocin), 136

T

Taclonex (calcipotriene/
 betamethasone
 dipropionate), 25
Tagamet (cimetidine), 36
Tagamet HB (cimetidine), 36
Tambocor (flecainide), 75
Tamiflu (oseltamivir), 133
TAO (troleandomycin), 178
Tapazole (methimazole), 113
Tarceva (erlotinib), 59
Targretin (bexarotene), 20
Tarka (trandolapril/verapamil),
 175
Tasigna (nilotinib), 126
Tasmar (tolcapone), 173
Taxol (paclitaxel), 136
Tazidime (ceftazidime), 31
Tazorac (tazarotene), 165
Taztia XT (diltiazem), 51

Teczem (diltiazem/enalapril),
 51
Tegison (etretinate), 72
Tegretol (carbamazepine), 27
Tekturna (aliskiren), 5
Tekturna HCT (aliskiren/HCTZ),
 5
Temodar (temozolomide), 166
Temovate (clobetasol), 39
Tempra (acetaminophen), 2
Tenex (guanfacine), 86
Tenoretic (atenolol/
 chlorthalidone), 14
Tenormin (atenolol), 14
Terazol-3 (terconazole), 167
Terazol-7 (terconazole), 167
Terazosin (terazosin), 167
Tessalon Perles (benzonatate),
 18
Testim (testosterone, topical),
 168
Tetracyn (tetracycline), 168
Thalitone (chlorthalidone), 35
Thalomid (thalidomide), 169
Theo-Dur (theophylline), 169
Thorazine (chlorpromazine), 35
Tiazac (diltiazem), 51
Ticar (ticarcillin), 170
Ticlid (ticlopidine), 171
Tikosyn (dofetilide), 53
Tilade (nedocromil), 125
Timentin (ticarcillin/clavulanate
 potassium), 170
Timolide (timolol/HCTZ), 171
Timoptic (timolol, ocular), 171

Tindamax (tinidazole), 172
TNKase (tenecteplase), 166
TobraDex (tobramycin/
    dexamethasone, ocular), 173
Tobrex (tobramycin, ocular), 172
Tofranil (imipramine HCl), 91
Tofranil-PM (imipramine
    pamoate), 92
Tolectin (tolmetin), 174
Tolinase (tolazamide), 173
Tonocard (tocainide), 173
Topamax (topiramate), 174
Toprol-XL (metoprolol), 116
Toradol (ketorolac), 99
Torisel (temsirolimus), 166
Tornalate (bitolterol), 21
Totacillin (ampicillin), 11
Tracleer (bosentan), 21
Trandate (labetalol), 99
Transderm-Nitro (nitroglycerin,
    transdermal), 128
Transderm-Scop
    (scopolamine), 159
Tranxene (clorazepate), 40
Travatan Z (travoprost), 176
Trazodone (trazodone), 176
Treanda (bendamustine), 18
Trecator-SC (ethionamide), 71
Trelstar Depot (triptorelin
    pamoate), 178
Trelstar LA (triptorelin
    pamoate), 178
Trental (pentoxifylline), 141
Trexall (methotrexate), 113
Treximet (sumatriptan/
    naproxen), 164
Triavil (perphenazine/
    amitriptyline), 141
TriCor (fenofibrate), 73
Tridesilon (desonide), 47
Tridil (nitroglycerin, injection),
    127
Triglide (fenofibrate), 73
Trilafon (perphenazine), 141
Trileptal (oxcarbazepine), 134
Tri-Levlen (ethinyl estradiol/
    levonorgestrel), 68
Trimox (amoxicillin), 9
Tri-Norinyl (ethinyl estradiol/
    norethindrone), 70
Triostat (liothyronine), 105
Triphasil (ethinyl estradiol/
    levonorgestrel), 68
Trisenox (arsenic trioxide), 13
Trivora-28 (ethinyl estradiol/
    levonorgestrel), 68
Trizivir (abacavir/lamivudine/
    zidovudine), 1
Trusopt (dorzolamide), 54
Truvada (tenofovir/
    emtricitabine), 167
Tussionex Pennkinetic
    (hydrocodone/
    chlorpheniramine), 88
Tusstat (diphenhydramine), 51
Tygacil (tigecycline), 171
Tykerb (lapatinib), 101
Tylenol (acetaminophen), 2
Tylox (oxycodone/
    acetaminophen), 135

Tysabri (natalizumab), 124
Tyzeka (telbivudine), 165

U

Ultracet (tramadol/
  acetaminophen), 175
Ultram (tramadol), 175
Ultram ER (tramadol), 175
Unasyn (ampicillin sodium/
  sulbactam sodium), 11
Unipen (nafcillin), 123
Uniretic (moexipril/HCTZ), 120
Univasc (moexipril), 120
Uroxatral (alfuzosin), 4
Urso (ursodiol), 179

V

Valcyte (valganciclovir), 179
Valisone (betamethasone
  valerate), 19
Valium (diazepam), 48
Valtrex (valacyclovir), 179
Vancenase (beclomethasone,
  nasal), 17
Vancenase AQ
  (beclomethasone, nasal), 17
Vanceril (beclomethasone,
  inhaled), 17
Vancocin (vancomycin), 180
Vancoled (vancomycin), 180
Vanos (fluocinonide), 76
Vantin (cefpodoxime), 31
Vaprisol (conivaptan), 42
Vascor (bepridil), 19
Vaseretic (enalapril/HCTZ), 57

Vasocon (naphazoline), 124
Vasotec (enalapril), 57
Vasotec IV (enalapril), 57
Vectibix (panitumumab), 137
Vectrin (minocycline), 119
Veetids (penicillin VK), 140
Velban (vinblastine), 182
Velcade (bortezomib), 21
Velosef (cephradine), 32
Ventavis (iloprost), 91
Ventolin HFA (albuterol), 3
Veramyst (fluticasone, nasal),
  78
Verdeso (desonide), 47
Veregen (sinecatechins,
  topical), 161
Verelan (verapamil), 181
Verelan PM (verapamil), 181
Vergon (meclizine), 110
Versed (midazolam), 118
VESIcare (solifenacin
  succinate), 162
Vexol (rimexolone), 155
VFEND (voriconazole), 182
Viagra (sildenafil), 160
Vibramycin (doxycycline), 54
Vibra-Tabs (doxycycline), 54
Vidaza (azacitidine), 15
Videx (didanosine [ddl]), 50
Videx EC (didanosine [ddl]), 50
Vigamox (moxifloxacin, ocular),
  122
Vincasar PFS (vincristine), 182
Vira-A (vidarabine), 181
Viracept (nelfinavir), 125

Viramune (nevirapine), 126
Virazole (ribavirin, aerosol), 154
Viread (tenofovir), 167
Viroptic (trifluridine), 178
Vision Blue (trypan blue), 179
Visken (pindolol), 143
Vistaril (hydroxyzine), 90
Vitamin B-12 (cyanocobalamin), 42
Vitrase (hyaluronidase, ovine), 87
Vivactil (protriptyline), 150
Vivelle (estradiol, transdermal), 62
Vivelle-Dot (estradiol, transdermal), 62
Vivitrol (naltrexone), 123
Voltaren (diclofenac, ocular), 49
Voltaren (diclofenac, oral), 49
Voltaren-XR (diclofenac, oral), 49
Vusion (miconazole/zinc oxide/white petrolatum), 118
Vytorin (ezetimibe/simvastatin), 73
Vyvanse (lisdexamfetamine dimesylate), 105

desiccated), 170
Wycillin (penicillin G procaine), 140
Wygesic (propoxyphene/acetaminophen), 148
Wymox (amoxicillin), 9
Wytensin (guanabenz), 85

X

Xalatan (latanoprost), 101
Xanax (alprazolam), 6
Xanax XR (alprazolam), 6
Xeloda (capecitabine), 26
Xenazine (tetrabenazine), 168
Xenical (orlistat), 133
Xibrom (bromfenac), 23
Xifaxan (rifaximin), 155
Xigris (drotrecogin alfa), 55
Xolair (omalizumab), 132
Xolegel (ketoconazole), 98
Xopenox (levalbuterol), 102
Xopenox HFA (levalbuterol), 102
Xylocaine (lidocaine), 104
Xyntha (antihemophilic factor), 12
Xyrem (oxybate, sodium), 134
Xyzal (levocetirizine), 103

W

Welchol (colesevelam), 41
Wellbutrin (bupropion), 24
Wellbutrin SR (bupropion), 24
Wellbutrin XL (bupropion), 24
Westhroid (thyroid

Y

Yasmin (ethinyl estradiol/drospirenone), 65
Yaz (ethinyl estradiol/drospirenone), 66
Yodoxin (iodoquinol), 96

Z

Zaditor (ketotifen), 99

Zagam (sparfloxacin), 162

Zanaflex (tizanidine), 172

Zantac 75 (ranitidine), 152

Zantac EFFERdose (ranitidine), 152

Zantac GELdose (ranitidine), 152

Zantryl (phentermine), 142

Zarontin (ethosuximide), 71

Zaroxolyn (metolazone), 116

Zavesca (miglustat), 119

Zebeta (bisoprolol), 21

Zefazone (cefmetazole), 30

Zegerid (omeprazole/sodium bicarbonate), 133

Zelapar (selegiline), 159

Zemplar (paricalcitol), 137

Zerit (stavudine [d4T]), 163

Zestoretic (lisinopril/HCTZ), 106

Zestril (lisinopril), 106

Zetia (ezetimibe), 72

Zevalin (ibritumomab), 90

Ziac (bisoprolol/HCTZ), 21

Ziagen (abacavir), 1

Zinacef (cefuroxime sodium), 32

Zingo (lidocaine), 104

Zithromax (azithromycin), 16

Zmax (azithromycin), 16

Zn-DTPA (pentetate zinc trisodium), 140

Zocor (simvastatin), 161

Zofran (ondansetron), 133

Zolinza (vorinostat), 182

Zoloft (sertraline), 160

Zometa (zoledronic acid), 184

Zomig (zolmitriptan), 184

Zomig-ZMT (zolmitriptan), 184

Zonalon (doxepin, topical), 54

Zonegran (zonisamide), 185

ZORprin (aspirin), 13

Zostavax (zoster vaccine), 185

Zosyn (piperacillin/ tazobactam), 144

Zovia 1/35E (ethinyl estradiol/ ethynodiol), 66

Zovia 1/50E (ethinyl estradiol/ ethynodiol), 66

Zovirax (acyclovir), 2

Zyban (bupropion), 24

Zyflo CR (zileuton), 184

Zylet (loteprednol/tobramycin), 108

Zyloprim (allopurinol), 5

Zymar (gatifloxacin, ocular), 83

Zyprexa (olanzapine), 131

Zyrtec (cetirizine), 33

Zyrtec-D (cetirizine/ pseudoephedrine), 33

Zyvox (linezolid), 105